Hom

Secrets of Our Ancestors

Discover the Long-Lost Herbal Remedies and Natural Cures of Our Past Generations

NOTICE: You <u>Do NOT</u> Have the Right to Reprint or Resell this Report

Disclaimer and/or Legal Notices:

While every attempt has been made to verify the information provided in this publication, neither the Author nor the Publisher assumes any responsibility for errors, omissions, or contrary interpretation of the subject matter herein. This publication is not intended for use as a source of legal or accounting advice. The Publisher wants to stress that the information contained herein may be subject to varying state and/or local laws or regulations. All users are advised to retain competent counsel to determine what state and/or local laws or regulations may apply to the user's particular business.

The Purchaser or Reader of this publication assumes responsibility for the use of these materials and information. Adherence to all applicable laws and regulations, federal, state, and local, governing professional licensing, business practices, advertising, and all other aspects of doing business in the United States or any other jurisdiction is the sole responsibility of the Purchaser or Reader. The Author and Publisher assume no responsibility or liability whatsoever on the behalf of any Purchaser or Reader of these materials. Any perceived slights of specific people or organizations are unintentional.

Health Disclaimer

The information contained in this book about home remedies is for general information purposes only. The information is not intended to be a substitute for professional medical advice, diagnosis, or treatment. Always seek the advice of a qualified healthcare provider with any questions you may have regarding a medical condition.

The remedies and techniques discussed in this book are not intended to diagnose, treat, cure, or prevent any disease. The results of using these remedies may vary from person to person and are not guaranteed.

It is important to remember that not all natural remedies are safe for everyone, and some may interact with medications or underlying health conditions. Before trying any natural remedy, it is recommended that you consult with a qualified healthcare provider to determine if it is appropriate for you.

This book is not intended to replace professional medical advice, and the author and publisher make no representations or warranties of any kind with respect to the accuracy, completeness, or suitability of the information contained in this book. The author and publisher will not be liable for any damages arising from the use or reliance on the information contained in this book.

This disclaimer applies to the entire content of this book and by using this information, the reader agrees to hold the author and publisher harmless from any and all liabilities.

WHAT ARE THE DIFFERENT TYPES OF NATURAL REMEDIES?

Natural remedies have been used for centuries to treat a variety of common ailments, serving as a safe and effective alternative to conventional medicine and prescription drugs. These remedies are made from natural ingredients such as herbs, spices, fruits, and vegetables, and are often prepared in the form of teas, salves, poultices, decoctions, and tinctures.

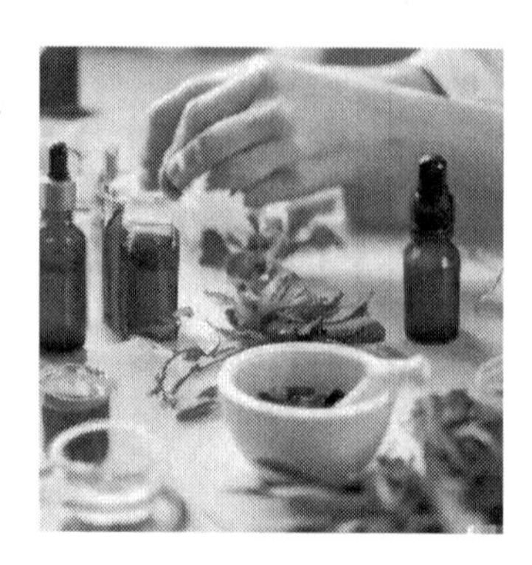

TEAS

Made from the leaves, flowers, roots, or seeds of plants, teas are a simple, effective, and accessible way to treat a variety of common ailments.

Stress and anxiety: Herbs such as chamomile, lavender, and passionflower have been shown to have calming and relaxing properties that can help to reduce stress and anxiety. Drinking a cup of tea made from these herbs can help to soothe the mind and body.

Insomnia: Herbs such as valerian root, passionflower, and chamomile have been used for centuries to treat insomnia and other sleep disorders, as they help to promote deep and restful sleep.

Digestive problems: Herbs such as ginger, peppermint, and fennel have been shown to have anti-inflammatory and antispasmodic properties, making them effective in treating digestive problems such as indigestion, nausea, and cramps.

Colds and flu: Herbs such as echinacea, elderberry, and ginger have been used for centuries to boost the immune system and treat colds and flu. These herbs are thought to have antiviral and antibacterial properties, helping to fight off infection and reduce symptoms such as cough, congestion, and fever.

Headaches: Herbs such as willow bark, feverfew, and ginger have been used to treat headaches and migraines. These herbs are thought to have pain-relieving and anti-inflammatory properties, helping to reduce headache pain and prevent migraines.

SALVES

Made from a combination of herbs, oils, and waxes, salves are applied topically to the skin to treat a variety of common ailments.

Skin conditions: Salves made from herbs such as calendula, comfrey, and plantain can be effective in treating skin conditions such as eczema, psoriasis, and rashes. These herbs have anti-inflammatory and healing properties that can help to soothe and heal irritated skin.

Muscle and joint pain: Salves made from herbs such as arnica, ginger, and turmeric can be effective in treating muscle and joint pain. These herbs have anti-inflammatory properties that can help to reduce pain and swelling, promoting faster recovery and improved mobility.

Cuts and wounds: Salves made from herbs such as calendula, comfrey, and yarrow can be effective in treating cuts and wounds. These herbs have antiseptic and healing properties that can help to prevent infection and promote faster healing.

Headaches: Salves made from herbs such as peppermint, lavender, and ginger can be effective in treating headaches. These herbs have pain-relieving and soothing properties that can help to reduce headache pain and tension.

Cold sores and other infections: Salves made from herbs such as tea tree, echinacea, and goldenseal can be effective in treating cold sores and other infections. These herbs have antiviral and antibacterial properties that can help to prevent and treat infections.

POULTICES

Poultices are an ancient form of herbal remedy that have been used for centuries as an alternative to traditional medicine and drugs. A poultice is a soft, moist mass of herbs and other materials that is applied directly to the skin to treat a variety of common ailments.

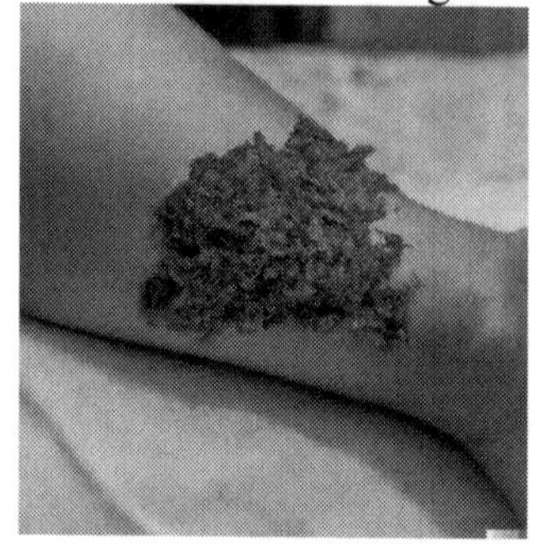

Inflammation and swelling: Poultices made from herbs such as turmeric, ginger, and plantain can be effective in reducing inflammation and swelling. These herbs have anti-inflammatory properties that can help to soothe and heal irritated skin.

Muscle and joint pain: Poultices made from herbs such as arnica, ginger, and comfrey can be effective in treating muscle and joint pain. These herbs have pain-relieving and anti-inflammatory properties that can help to reduce pain and swelling, promoting faster recovery and improved mobility.

Cuts and wounds: Poultices made from herbs such as yarrow, comfrey, and calendula can be effective in treating cuts and wounds. These herbs have antiseptic and healing properties that can help to prevent infection and promote faster healing.

Chest congestion: Poultices made from herbs such as eucalyptus, menthol, and thyme can be effective in treating chest congestion. These herbs have expectorant and decongestant properties that can help to loosen mucus and relieve respiratory symptoms.

Headaches: Poultices made from herbs such as peppermint, lavender, and ginger can be effective in treating headaches. These herbs have pain-relieving and soothing properties that can help to reduce headache pain and tension.

DECOCTIONS

A decoction is a concentrated liquid extract made by boiling herbs in water and is typically taken orally to treat a variety of common ailments.

Digestive issues: Decoctions made from herbs such as ginger, fennel, and peppermint can be effective in treating digestive issues such as nausea, indigestion, and bloating. These herbs have carminative properties that can help to soothe the digestive tract and promote healthy digestion.

Respiratory issues: Decoctions made from herbs such as thyme, eucalyptus, and mullein can be effective in treating respiratory issues such as bronchitis, congestion, and coughing. These herbs have expectorant and decongestant properties that can help to loosen mucus and relieve respiratory symptoms.

Stress and anxiety: Decoctions made from herbs such as valerian, passionflower, and kava can be effective in treating stress and anxiety. These herbs have sedative and calming properties that can help to promote relaxation and reduce feelings of stress and anxiety.

Insomnia: Decoctions made from herbs such as chamomile, valerian, and passionflower can be effective in treating insomnia. These herbs have sedative properties that can help to promote sleep and improve the quality of rest.

Immune system support: Decoctions made from herbs such as echinacea, astragalus, and elderberry can be effective in boosting the immune system. These herbs have immune-boosting properties that can help to prevent and treat infections.

TINCTURES

Tinctures are made by soaking herbs in alcohol or vinegar, and the resulting liquid extract is then taken orally to treat a variety of common ailments.

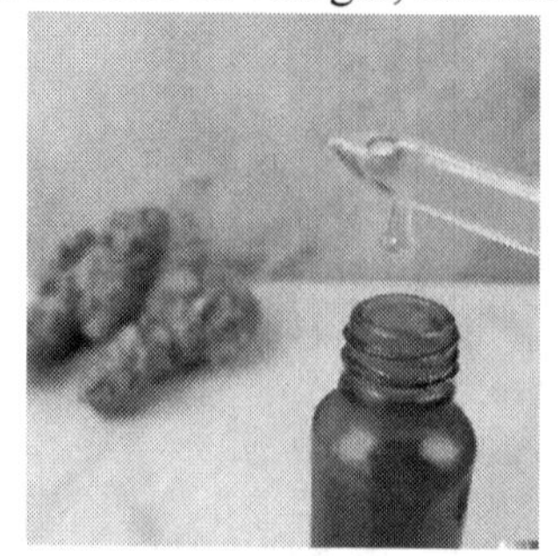

Digestive issues: Tinctures made from herbs such as ginger, fennel, and peppermint can be effective in treating digestive issues such as nausea, indigestion, and bloating. These herbs have carminative properties that can help to soothe the digestive tract and promote healthy digestion.

Respiratory issues: Tinctures made from herbs such as thyme, eucalyptus, and mullein can be effective in treating respiratory issues such as bronchitis, congestion, and coughing. These herbs have expectorant and decongestant properties that can help to loosen mucus and relieve respiratory symptoms.

Stress and anxiety: Tinctures made from herbs such as valerian, passionflower, and kava can be effective in treating stress and anxiety. These herbs have sedative and calming properties that can help to promote relaxation and reduce feelings of stress and anxiety.

Insomnia: Tinctures made from herbs such as chamomile, valerian, and passionflower can be effective in treating insomnia. These herbs have sedative properties that can help to promote sleep and improve the quality of rest.

Immune system support: Tinctures made from herbs such as echinacea, astragalus, and elderberry can be effective in boosting the immune system. These herbs have immune-boosting properties that can help to prevent and treat infections.

In addition to these common types of natural remedies, there are also many other methods used to treat common ailments, such as aromatherapy, acupuncture, and homeopathy.

AROMATHERAPY

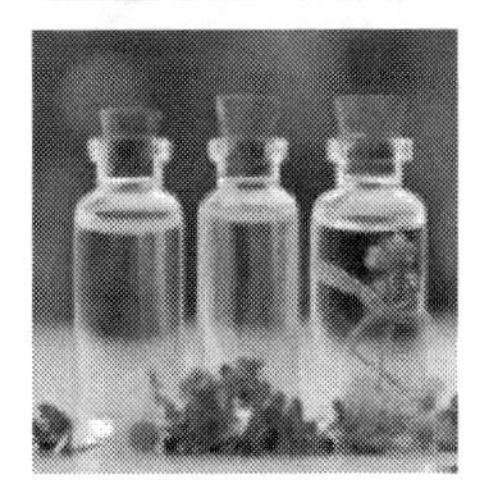

Aromatherapy involves the use of essential oils to treat various health conditions.

Essential oils are extracted from plants and have been used for centuries to promote relaxation, alleviate pain, and improve mood.

ACUPUNCTURE

Acupuncture is a traditional Chinese medicine technique that involves the insertion of fine needles into specific points on the body to stimulate the flow of energy and improve health.

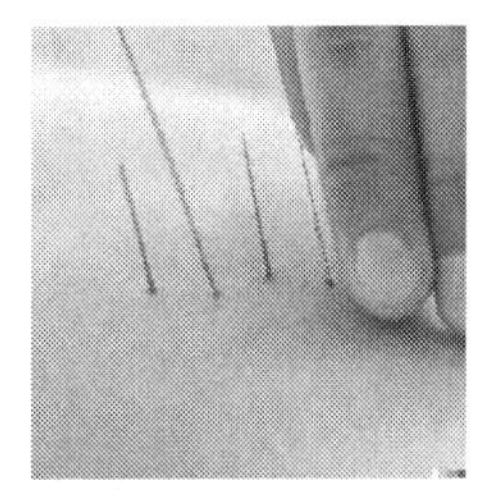

HOMEOPATHY

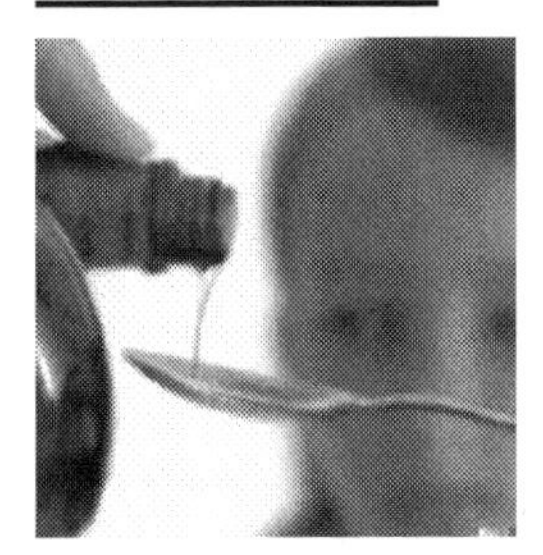

Homeopathy is a holistic medical system that uses highly diluted substances to stimulate the body's natural healing process.

Homeopathic remedies are often used to treat conditions such as allergies, headaches, and insomnia.

REMEDIES FOR COMMON AILMENTS

In this chapter we're going to cover many of the common ailments. Some of these ailments can be treated by modern medicine with antibiotics, antivirals or other medications while others there are limited medicines available. The natural remedies we cover are tried and true and have been used by people all over the world for hundreds or even thousands of years.

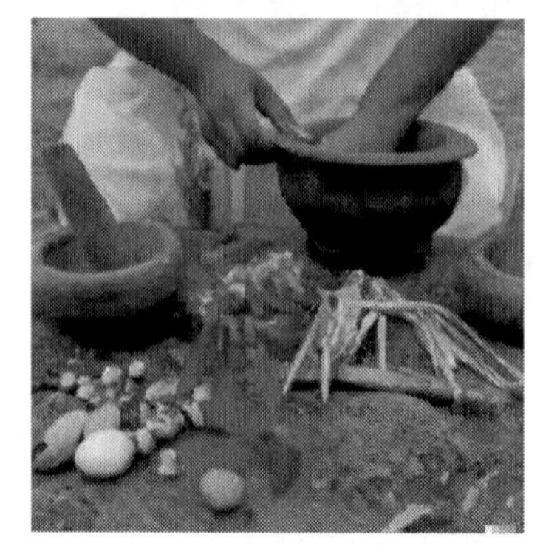

It's important to keep in mind that these remedies are not a substitute for proper medical treatment, and you should always see a doctor if the remedies are not working or your condition is life threatening.

However, they can be used in conjunction with antibiotics or other modern medicine treatments to help alleviate the symptoms and speed up the healing process. As with any natural remedy, it's always best to talk to your doctor before trying something new, especially if you have any pre-existing health conditions.

ALLERGIES & HAY FEVER

Seasonal allergies can be a major source of discomfort for many people, causing symptoms such as sneezing, runny nose, and itching eyes.

Local honey: Consuming local honey is thought to contain trace amounts of pollen from local plants, which can help desensitize your immune system to allergens.

Saline nasal rinse: Rinsing your nasal passages with a saline solution can help remove allergens and relieve congestion.

Butterbur: Butterbur is a herb that can reduce symptoms such as sneezing, runny nose, and itching eyes.

Quercetin: Quercetin is a natural antioxidant that is found in many fruits and vegetables and has been shown to have anti-inflammatory effects.

Nettles: Nettles contain histamine, which can help reduce allergy symptoms. Nettles can be taken in supplement form or used in teas.

Ginger: Ginger has anti-inflammatory properties that can help reduce sneezing and runny nose. Ginger can be taken in supplement form or used fresh in cooking and teas.

Vitamin C: Vitamin C is a natural antihistamine that can help reduce allergy symptoms, such as sneezing and runny nose.

ANEMIA

Anemia is a condition in which the body does not have enough red blood cells, which can lead to fatigue, weakness, and decreased overall health.

Iron-rich foods: Some of the best iron-rich foods include red meat, poultry, fish, beans, lentils, and dark leafy greens such as spinach and kale.

Vitamin C: Vitamin C can help improve the absorption of iron from the foods you eat. Foods high in vitamin C include oranges, strawberries, bell peppers, and broccoli.

Folic acid: Folic acid is a B vitamin that is important to produce red blood cells. Foods high in folic acid include leafy greens, beans, lentils, and citrus fruits.

Herbs: Yellow dock root, dandelion root, and alfalfa.

ARTHRITIS

Arthritis is a common condition that affects millions of people worldwide and causes inflammation, pain, and stiffness in the joints.

Ginger contains compounds called gingerols and shogaols that have anti-inflammatory properties and can help reduce swelling and pain in the joints. You can consume ginger in the form of tea, supplements, or by adding it to your food.

Turmeric has been shown to be effective in reducing joint pain and swelling in people with arthritis. You can consume turmeric in the form of a supplement or add it to your food.

Devil's Claw is an herb with anti-inflammatory properties that can help reduce swelling and stiffness in the joints. Devil's Claw is available in supplement form or as a tea.

Willow Bark contains compounds similar to aspirin and has been shown to be effective in reducing joint pain and swelling. You can find Willow Bark in supplement form or as a tea.

Boswellia has anti-inflammatory properties and can help reduce swelling and stiffness in the joints. Available in supplement form or as a resin that can be used in a tea or applied topically.

Glucosamine and Chondroitin are natural compounds that are found in the cartilage of joints and are effective in reducing joint pain and improving joint health. Glucosamine and Chondroitin are available in supplement form and can be taken orally.

ASTHMA

Asthma is a chronic condition that affects the airways, causing wheezing, shortness of breath, and chest tightness.

Butterbur: Butterbur has been shown to help reduce the frequency and severity of asthma symptoms, such as wheezing and shortness of breath. It is believed to reduce airway inflammation and relax the muscles that surround the airways.

Ginger: Ginger has anti-inflammatory properties that can help reduce airway inflammation and relieve asthma symptoms.

Turmeric: Turmeric is a spice that contains curcumin, which has anti-inflammatory properties that can help reduce airway inflammation and relieve asthma symptoms. Turmeric can be taken in supplement form or used fresh in cooking.

Bromelain: Bromelain is a substance found in pineapples that has anti-inflammatory properties that can help reduce airway inflammation and relieve asthma symptoms.

BACK PAIN

Back pain is a common complaint, affecting millions of people worldwide. Fortunately, there are quite a few natural options for treating it at home.

Exercise: Gentle exercises such as yoga, stretching, and low-impact activities like swimming or cycling can help strengthen the muscles in the back and reduce pain.

Heat therapy: Applying heat to the affected area, such as a warm towel or heating pad, can help relax tight muscles and relieve pain.

Massage: Massaging the affected area can help improve circulation and reduce muscle tension, leading to less pain.

Willow bark: Willow bark contains salicin, which is converted into salicylic acid in the body and acts as a natural pain reliever.

Ginger: Ginger has anti-inflammatory properties that can help reduce pain and swelling in the back.

Turmeric: Turmeric has anti-inflammatory properties that have been used to treat a variety of conditions, including back pain.

Devil's claw: This herb is native to southern Africa and has been used to treat back pain, as well as other joint pain and inflammation.

Arnica: Arnica is a plant that is used to relieve pain, swelling, and stiffness. It is available in creams, ointments, and tinctures.

BOILS

Boils are painful skin infections that occur when bacteria infect a hair follicle or oil gland. Here are some of the most used natural remedies and herbs for treating boils.

Tea tree oil: Tea tree oil has antibacterial properties that can help kill the bacteria that cause boils. Apply a small amount of the oil directly to the affected area using a cotton swab.

Echinacea: Echinacea is an herb that has been used for centuries to boost the immune system and fight infections.

Garlic: Garlic has antibacterial and antiviral properties that can help kill the bacteria that cause boils.

Turmeric: Turmeric is a spice that contains curcumin, which can help reduce swelling and pain associated with boils.

BUG BITES & STINGS

Bug bites and stings can be a nuisance and can cause discomfort, itching, and swelling. While most bug bites and stings are relatively harmless, some people may experience an allergic reaction.

Aloe vera: Aloe vera is a plant that has been used for centuries to soothe skin and reduce itching and swelling. Apply the gel directly to the affected area.

Tea tree oil: Tea tree oil has antibacterial properties that can help prevent infection and reduce itching and swelling. Apply a small amount of the oil directly to the affected area using a cotton swab.

Lavender oil: Lavender oil has calming and soothing properties to reduce itching and swelling from bug bites & stings. Apply a small amount of the oil to the affected area using a cotton swab.

Echinacea: Echinacea is an herb that has been used for centuries to boost the immune system and fight infections.

BURNS

Burns can be caused by a variety of factors, including heat, chemicals, radiation, and electricity. Burns can be painful and cause redness, blistering, and itching. While mild burns can often be treated at home with over-the-counter creams, more severe burns may require medical attention. Let's look at some of the most popular natural remedies and herbs for treating burns.

Aloe vera: Aloe vera has been used for centuries to soothe skin and reduce itching and pain. To use aloe vera for burns, simply apply the gel directly to the affected area.

Honey: Honey has antibacterial properties that can help prevent infection and promote healing. To use honey for burns, apply a thin layer of honey to the affected area and cover with a bandage.

Tea tree oil: Tea tree oil has antibacterial properties that can help prevent infection and reduce itching and pains. Apply a small amount of the oil directly to the affected area using a cotton swab.

Calendula: Calendula has anti-inflammatory and antibacterial properties that can help soothe skin and reduce itching and pain associated with burns.

BURSITIS

Bursitis is a condition that occurs when the bursae, small fluid-filled sacs that cushion the bones and muscles, become inflamed.

This condition can cause pain, swelling, and stiffness in the affected joint. Bursitis is often caused by overuse, injury, or an underlying medical condition such as rheumatoid arthritis.

Turmeric: Curcumin, a compound found in turmeric, has been shown to reduce inflammation in the body and may be effective in treating bursitis.

Ginger is another spice with anti-inflammatory and pain-relieving properties. You can take it in supplement form or add it to your diet in the form of a tea or spice.

Boswellia is an herb that has anti-inflammatory and pain-relieving properties. Take it in supplement form or use it in a topical cream.

Willow bark is an herb that has pain-relieving properties. Take it in supplement form or use it in a topical cream.

CANKER & COLD SORES

Canker sores and cold sores are common skin conditions that can cause pain, discomfort, and embarrassment.

Aloe Vera: To use Aloe Vera for canker sores or cold sores, you can apply the gel directly to the affected area several times a day.

Licorice is an herb that has been used for centuries to treat canker sores and cold sores. You can take it in supplement form or apply a licorice-based ointment to the affected area.

Tea tree oil has antiseptic and anti-inflammatory properties. Dilute the oil with a carrier oil and apply it directly to the affected area.

L-Lysine is an amino acid that can help reduce the frequency and severity of canker and cold sores. Take it in supplement form.

Alum is a natural astringent that can help dry out the sores and reduce pain and swelling. Apply directly to the sore using a cotton swab or mix with water and rinse over the affected area.

Baking Soda has a neutralizing effect on the pH levels and can help reduce discomfort. Mix with water to form a paste and apply directly to the sore or use during teeth brushing.

COLD & FLU

The common cold and flu are two of the most widespread illnesses that affect millions of people each year. Symptoms such as runny nose, cough, headache, fatigue, and muscle aches can make you feel miserable for several days.

Garlic is an antiviral and antibacterial agent that can help fight cold and flu viruses. It can be consumed raw, cooked or in supplements.

Ginger has anti-inflammatory properties that help relieve headaches, congestion, and sore throat. You can take it in supplement form or add it to your diet in the form of a tea or spice.

Echinacea has antiviral and antibacterial properties that can help fight off viruses and bacteria that cause cold and flu.

Honey is a cough suppressant that can help soothe a sore throat. It can be consumed alone or mixed with lemon juice and hot water.

Elderberry is high in antioxidants and has antiviral properties that can help reduce symptoms such as congestion, cough, and fever. Elderberry can be consumed in supplement form or as a syrup.

Vitamin C: Supplements or foods high in Vitamin C, such as oranges, lemon, and kiwi, can help boost the immune system and reduce the severity of cold and flu symptoms.

Chicken soup: Chicken soup has been a traditional remedy for cold and flu for centuries. The hot liquid can relieve congestion, while the nutrients in the chicken can help boost the immune system.

COLITIS AND CROHN'S DISEASE

Colitis and Crohn's Disease are two types of Inflammatory Bowel Diseases (IBD) that can cause discomfort and affect your daily life. Symptoms such as abdominal pain, diarrhea, and rectal bleeding can be debilitating and make it difficult to manage daily activities. While there is no cure for these conditions, natural remedies and herbs can help alleviate symptoms and improve quality of life.

Aloe Vera can help reduce inflammation in the intestines and alleviate symptoms such as abdominal pain and diarrhea. It can be taken in supplement form or applied topically.

Ginger has been shown to be effective in reducing symptoms of colitis and Crohn's Disease. It has anti-inflammatory properties that can help reduce inflammation in the intestines and alleviate symptoms such as abdominal pain and diarrhea.

Turmeric: Turmeric has been shown to be effective in reducing symptoms of colitis and Crohn's Disease.

Probiotics are beneficial bacteria that maintain a healthy gut, and have been shown to reduce symptoms of colitis and Crohn's. They come in supplement form or found in foods such as yogurt and kefir.

Omega-3 fatty acids: Omega-3 fatty acids are essential fatty acids that can help reduce inflammation in the body. They can be found in supplement form or in fatty fish such as salmon and mackerel.

Psyllium: Psyllium is a type of soluble fiber that can help regulate bowel movements and reduce symptoms of diarrhea. Psyllium can be consumed in supplement form or added to food as a thickener.

Fasting: During fasting, the digestive system is given a break, allowing it to rest and heal. Fasting should only be done under the guidance of a healthcare provider.

CONJUNCTIVITIS (PINK EYE)

Conjunctivitis, also known as "pink eye," is a common eye condition characterized by redness, itching, and discharge in the eye. It can be caused by a variety of factors, including bacteria, viruses, allergies, or irritants.

Warm compresses: Applying a warm compress to the affected eye can help to reduce inflammation and relieve discomfort. Simply soak a clean cloth in warm water, wring it out, and hold it over the affected eye for a few minutes. Repeat as needed.

Tea bags: Used tea bags can be used as a warm compress for treating conjunctivitis. The tannins in the tea have anti-inflammatory properties and can help to soothe the eye.

Honey has antibacterial properties and can help to soothe the eye and reduce inflammation. Mix a small amount of honey with warm water and apply the mixture to a clean cloth. Hold the cloth over the affected eye for a few minutes.

Aloe Vera has anti-inflammatory and moisturizing properties that can help to soothe the eye. Apply a small amount of Aloe Vera gel to a clean cloth and hold it over the affected eye for a few minutes.

Chamomile is an anti-inflammatory herb that can help to soothe the eye. Steep a chamomile tea bag in warm water for a few minutes, remove the tea bag, and let it cool to a comfortable temperature. Hold the tea bag over the affected eye for a few minutes.

Calendula is an anti-inflammatory herb that can help to soothe the eye. Steep calendula flowers in hot water for a few minutes, remove the flowers, and let the liquid cool to a comfortable temperature. Use a clean cloth to apply the liquid to the affected eye.

CONSTIPATION

Constipation is a common digestive issue that affects millions of people worldwide. It is characterized by infrequent bowel movements, hard and dry stools, and discomfort during elimination.

Fiber is essential for healthy bowel movements and preventing constipation. Foods include whole grains, fruits, and vegetables.

Hydration is essential for preventing constipation. Aim to drink at least 8 glasses of water per day to prevent constipation.

Prunes contain fiber and natural sugars that regulate bowel movements and soften stools. Eat prunes or drink prune juice.

Flaxseeds are rich in fiber and are effective in treating constipation. They help regulate bowel movements and soften stools.

Senna is a natural remedy for constipation. It works by stimulating the muscles in the intestines, promoting bowel movements.

Ginger has natural digestive properties that help regulate bowel movements and prevent constipation.

Castor Oil works by lubricating the intestines and promoting bowel movements. Castor oil should be taken on an empty stomach, as it can cause discomfort if taken after a meal.

COUGH

A persistent cough can be an annoyance and disrupt your daily life. It can be caused by a number of factors, including the common cold, bronchitis, and pneumonia.

Honey: Honey works by coating the throat and reducing irritation. Mix a teaspoon of honey with warm water or tea, or consume it directly for a natural way to treat a persistent cough.

Ginger: Ginger has anti-inflammatory properties that can help reduce inflammation in the throat and ease a persistent cough.

Marshmallow Root: Marshmallow root is a herb that has been used for centuries to treat coughs and other respiratory issues. It works by reducing irritation in the throat and promoting healing. Marshmallow root can be consumed as a tea or in supplement form.

Licorice Root: Licorice root has anti-inflammatory properties that can help reduce irritation in the throat and ease a persistent cough. It can be consumed as a tea or in supplement form.

Echinacea: Echinacea works by boosting the immune system and reducing inflammation in the respiratory system.

Thyme: Thyme is an herb that has antiseptic properties and can be used to treat a persistent cough. It works by reducing inflammation in the throat and promoting healing.

Steam: Steam helps to loosen mucus and soothe the throat, reducing irritation and easing a persistent cough. Simply add hot water to a bowl and inhale the steam or take a hot shower.

CUTS & BRUISES

Aloe Vera: Aloe Vera has antibacterial and anti-inflammatory properties that can help reduce redness, swelling, and discomfort.

Arnica: Arnica has anti-inflammatory properties that can help reduce swelling and discomfort. Arnica can be applied directly to the skin as a cream or ointment, or consumed in supplement form.

Witch Hazel: Witch Hazel works by reducing swelling and redness, and promoting healing. Witch hazel can be applied directly to the skin as a toner or astringent.

Calendula: Calendula has antibacterial and anti-inflammatory properties that promote healing and reduce redness and swelling. Calendula can be applied directly to the skin as a cream or ointment.

Turmeric: Turmeric can help reduce swelling and discomfort in cuts and bruises. Simply mix turmeric powder with a little water to make a paste and apply it directly to the affected area.

Tea Tree Oil: Tea Tree Oil is a natural antiseptic that works by reducing the risk of infection and promoting healing. Simply dilute tea tree oil with a carrier oil and apply it directly to the affected area.

Cold Compress: A cold compress can be an effective way to reduce swelling and discomfort in cuts and bruises. Wrap a bag of ice or a frozen vegetable in a towel and apply it directly for 10-15 minutes.

DANDRUFF

Dandruff and dry scalp are common skin conditions that can be uncomfortable, unsightly, and embarrassing.

Tea Tree Oil: Tea Tree Oil is a natural antifungal and antiseptic that has been used for centuries to treat dandruff and dry scalp. Simply dilute a few drops of tea tree oil with a carrier oil, such as coconut oil, and massage into the scalp. Leave on for a few minutes, then rinse with a gentle shampoo.

Apple Cider Vinegar: Apple Cider Vinegar is a natural astringent that has been used for centuries to treat dandruff and dry scalp. Simply mix equal parts water and apple cider vinegar, and massage into the scalp. Leave on for a few minutes, then rinse with water.

Aloe Vera: Aloe Vera is a natural moisturizer that can treat dandruff and dry scalp. Apply aloe vera gel directly to the scalp, and massage into the skin. Leave on for a few minutes, then rinse with water.

Coconut Oil: Coconut Oil is a natural moisturizer used to treat dandruff and dry scalp. Massage coconut oil into the scalp, and leave on for a few hours or overnight. Rinse with a gentle shampoo.

Baking Soda: Baking Soda is a natural exfoliant that has been used for centuries to treat dandruff and dry scalp. Simply mix baking soda with water to make a paste, and massage into the scalp. Leave on for a few minutes, then rinse with water.

Neem Oil: Neem Oil is a natural antifungal and antiseptic that has been used for centuries to treat dandruff and dry scalp. Simply massage neem oil into the scalp, and leave on for a few hours or overnight. Rinse with a gentle shampoo.

Lemon Juice: Lemon Juice is a natural astringent that has been used to treat dandruff and dry scalp. Simply massage lemon juice into the scalp, and leave on for a few minutes. Rinse with water.

DEMENTIA/MEMORY LOSS

Dementia and memory loss can be devastating conditions, leading to a decline in cognitive function and quality of life. While there is no cure for dementia, there are natural remedies and herbs that can help improve memory and slow down the progression of the disease.

Ginkgo Biloba: Ginkgo Biloba is an herb that improves memory and cognitive function. It is believed to increase blood flow to the brain, which can protect against brain damage and improve memory.

Turmeric: Turmeric has been shown to improve cognitive function and reduce the risk of developing dementia.

Bacopa: Bacopa is an herb that is commonly used in Ayurvedic medicine to improve memory and cognitive function. It has been shown to increase the production of brain chemicals that are associated with improved memory and cognitive function.

Rosemary: Rosemary is an herb known for its memory-enhancing properties. It has been shown to improve cognitive function and reduce the risk of developing dementia.

Omega-3 Fatty Acids: Omega-3 fatty acids are essential for brain health and have been shown to improve memory and cognitive function, as well as reduce the risk of developing dementia.

Exercise: Exercise has been shown to improve memory and cognitive function, as well as reduce the risk of developing dementia. Regular physical activity can help keep the brain healthy and functioning optimally.

DIABETES

Diabetes is a chronic condition that affects millions of people worldwide. It occurs when the body is unable to properly produce or use insulin, leading to high blood sugar levels. While there is no cure for diabetes, there are natural remedies and herbs that can help manage the condition and improve overall health.

Cinnamon: Cinnamon has been shown to improve insulin sensitivity and lower blood sugar levels in people with diabetes. It is believed to work by increasing the effectiveness of insulin and decreasing the amount of glucose produced by the liver.

Bitter Melon: Bitter melon is a vegetable that is known for its anti-diabetic properties. It has been shown to improve insulin sensitivity and lower blood sugar levels in people with diabetes.

Fenugreek: Fenugreek is an herb that has been used for centuries to manage diabetes. It has been shown to improve insulin sensitivity and lower blood sugar levels, as well as reduce the risk of developing diabetes-related complications.

Gymnema Sylvestre: Gymnema Sylvestre is an herb that has been used in Ayurvedic medicine to manage diabetes. It has been shown to improve insulin sensitivity and lower blood sugar levels, as well as reduce the risk of developing diabetes-related complications.

Alpha-Lipoic Acid: Alpha-lipoic acid is a powerful antioxidant that has been shown to improve insulin sensitivity and lower blood sugar levels in people with diabetes.

Magnesium: Magnesium is a mineral that has been shown to improve insulin sensitivity and lower blood sugar levels, as well as reduce the risk of developing diabetes-related complications.

Exercise: Exercise has been shown to improve insulin sensitivity and lower blood sugar levels in people with diabetes. Regular physical activity helps keep the body healthy and functioning.

DIARRHEA

Diarrhea is a common digestive problem that can be caused by a variety of factors such as food poisoning, viral infections, and certain medications. It is characterized by frequent loose or watery stools and can lead to dehydration if left untreated.

Ginger: Ginger has been used for centuries to treat digestive problems, including diarrhea. Its anti-inflammatory and antioxidant properties can help soothe an upset stomach and reduce inflammation in the gut.

Chamomile: Chamomile is a natural antispasmodic and has a calming effect on the digestive system. Drinking chamomile tea can help to reduce cramping, bloating, and diarrhea.

Peppermint: Peppermint's antispasmodic properties can help relax the muscles in the digestive tract and relieve cramping. You can drink peppermint tea or chew on fresh peppermint leaves.

Fennel: Fennel is a natural carminative, which means it can help to relieve bloating and gas. Drinking fennel tea or chewing on fresh fennel seeds can help soothe an upset stomach and reduce diarrhea.

Licorice: Licorice has a soothing effect on the digestive tract and can help to reduce inflammation and relieve symptoms.

Aloe Vera: Drinking aloe Vera juice can help to reduce inflammation in the gut and relieve symptoms of diarrhea.

Probiotics: Probiotics can help to maintain a healthy balance of gut bacteria. Taking a probiotic supplement can help to restore the balance of gut bacteria and relieve symptoms of diarrhea.

DIVERTICULITIS

Diverticulitis is a digestive condition that affects the colon and is characterized by the formation of small pockets (diverticula) in the colon wall. These pockets can become infected and inflamed, leading to a painful condition called diverticulitis.

Fiber-rich foods: A high-fiber diet can help by promoting regular bowel movements and reducing the risk of constipation. Foods rich in fiber include whole grains, fruits, and vegetables.

Probiotics: taking a probiotic supplement can help to restore the balance of gut bacteria and reduce the risk of diverticulitis.

Ginger: Ginger can help to soothe an upset stomach and reduce inflammation in the gut. Drinking ginger tea or chewing on a piece of fresh ginger can help to relieve symptoms of diverticulitis.

Turmeric: Taking turmeric supplements or adding turmeric to your diet can help to reduce inflammation and relieve symptoms of diverticulitis.

Slippery Elm: Slippery Elm is an herb that can help to soothe the digestive tract and reduce inflammation. Taking slippery elm tea or supplements can help to relieve symptoms of diverticulitis.

Aloe Vera: Aloe Vera is known for its anti-inflammatory and soothing properties. Drinking aloe Vera juice can help to reduce inflammation in the gut and relieve symptoms of diverticulitis.

Peppermint: Peppermint can help to relax the muscles in the digestive tract and relieve cramping. Drinking peppermint tea or chewing fresh peppermint leaves can help to relieve diverticulitis.

EAR PAIN / EARACHE

Earaches can be a debilitating condition that affects people of all ages. The pain and discomfort can be intense and make it difficult to perform everyday tasks.

Garlic Oil: To make garlic oil, simply heat a few garlic cloves in olive oil until they are fragrant. Strain the oil and let it cool to a comfortable temperature. Apply a few drops of the oil into the affected ear and let it sit for a few minutes. Repeat this process a few times a day until the pain subsides.

Onions: To use this remedy, chop an onion into small pieces and heat it in a pan until it begins to caramelize. Let the onion cool to a comfortable temperature and apply a few drops of the juice into the affected ear. Repeat this process a few times a day until the pain subsides.

Ginger: To use this remedy, steep a small piece of ginger in boiling water for 10 minutes. Strain the liquid and let it cool to a comfortable temperature. Apply a few drops of the liquid into the affected ear and let it sit for a few minutes. Repeat this process a few times a day until the pain subsides.

Echinacea: Steep a small handful of echinacea flowers and leaves in boiling water for 10 minutes. Strain the liquid and let it cool to a comfortable temperature. Apply a few drops of the liquid into affected ear and let sit for a few minutes. Repeat process a few times a day until pain subsides.

Mullein: Steep a small handful of mullein flowers and leaves in boiling water for 10 minutes. Strain the liquid and let it cool to a comfortable temperature. Apply a few drops of the liquid into the affected ear and let it sit for a few minutes. Repeat this process a few times a day until the pain subsides.

ECZEMA

Eczema, also known as atopic dermatitis, is a common skin condition characterized by dry, itchy, and inflamed skin. While there are several conventional treatments available, many people prefer to use natural remedies and herbs to treat this condition. Here are some of the most popular and effective natural remedies and herbs for treating eczema.

Aloe Vera: Aloe Vera has anti-inflammatory and moisturizing properties that can help to soothe dry and irritated skin. Applying aloe Vera gel directly to the skin can relieve symptoms of eczema.

Coconut oil: Coconut oil is a natural moisturizer that can help to hydrate dry skin and reduce inflammation. Applying coconut oil directly to the skin can help to relieve symptoms of eczema.

Oatmeal: Oatmeal can soothe dry and itchy skin. Adding oatmeal to your bath or making an oatmeal paste to apply directly to the skin can help to relieve symptoms of eczema.

Chamomile: Chamomile has a calming effect on the skin. Drinking chamomile tea or applying chamomile essential oil directly to the skin can help to relieve symptoms of eczema.

Tea tree oil: Tea tree oil is a natural antiseptic that can help to relieve symptoms of eczema. Dilute tea tree oil with a carrier oil such as coconut oil and apply directly to the skin.

Vitamin E: Vitamin E is a powerful antioxidant that can help to reduce inflammation and improve the health of the skin. Taking a vitamin E supplement or applying vitamin E oil directly to the skin can help to relieve symptoms of eczema.

FIBROMYALGIA

Fibromyalgia is a chronic condition characterized by widespread pain, tenderness, and fatigue. While there is no cure for fibromyalgia, there are several natural remedies and herbs that can help to relieve symptoms and improve quality of life.

Magnesium: Magnesium is a mineral that can help to reduce muscle pain and improve sleep. Taking a magnesium supplement or eating magnesium-rich foods can help to relieve symptoms.

Ginger: Ginger has anti-inflammatory and pain-relieving properties that can help to relieve symptoms of fibromyalgia. Drinking ginger tea or taking ginger supplements can help to reduce muscle pain..

Turmeric: Turmeric is a spice with powerful anti-inflammatory properties. Taking turmeric supplements or adding turmeric to your diet can help to reduce inflammation and relieve symptoms.

Willow bark: Willow bark is a pain reliever that contains salicin, a compound similar to aspirin. Taking willow bark supplements or drinking willow bark tea can help to relieve symptoms.

SAM-e: S-adenosylmethionine (SAM-e) is a naturally occurring compound that can help to relieve pain and improve mood. Taking SAM-e supplements can help to relieve symptoms of fibromyalgia.

GAS & BLOATING

Bloating and gas are common digestive complaints that can cause discomfort and embarrassment.

Peppermint: Peppermint is a natural antispasmodic that can help to relieve bloating. Drinking peppermint tea or taking peppermint oil capsules can soothe the digestive system and reduce bloating.

Fennel: Fennel is an antispasmodic and carminative. Drinking fennel tea or taking fennel supplements can soothe the digestive system and reduce symptoms of bloating and gas.

Ginger: Ginger is a natural anti-inflammatory and carminative. Drinking ginger tea or taking ginger supplements can help to soothe the digestive system and reduce symptoms of bloating and gas.

Probiotics: Probiotics are beneficial bacteria that can help to improve digestive health. Taking a probiotic supplement or consuming probiotic-rich foods such as yogurt and kefir can help to improve digestive health and reduce symptoms of bloating and gas.

Charcoal: Charcoal is a natural absorbent that can help to remove excess gas from the digestive system. Taking charcoal supplements or consuming activated charcoal can reduce bloating and gas.

Exercise: Regular exercise can help by improving digestion and promoting the release of gas from the digestive system. Engaging in moderate physical activity such as walking, cycling, or yoga can help to reduce symptoms of bloating and gas.

GOUT

Gout is a type of arthritis that causes pain and swelling in the joints. It is caused by a buildup of uric acid in the body, which forms crystals that deposit in the joints.

Cherries: Cherries are a natural anti-inflammatory. Eating a handful of cherries or drinking cherry juice can help to reduce inflammation and relieve pain in people with gout.

Ginger: Ginger is a natural anti-inflammatory. Drinking ginger tea or taking ginger supplements can help to reduce inflammation and relieve symptoms of gout.

Apple cider vinegar: Apple cider vinegar is an alkalizing agent that can reduce uric acid levels in the body. Drinking a mixture of apple cider vinegar and water can help to reduce symptoms of gout.

Vitamin C: Taking vitamin C supplements or consuming vitamin C-rich foods such as oranges, strawberries, and bell peppers can help to reduce inflammation and relieve symptoms of gout.

Devil's claw: Devil's claw is a natural anti-inflammatory. Taking devil's claw supplements or drinking devil's claw tea can help to reduce inflammation and relieve symptoms of gout.

Bromelain: Bromelain is a natural anti-inflammatory that can help to reduce pain and swelling in people with gout. Taking bromelain supplements or consuming bromelain-rich foods such as pineapples can help to reduce inflammation and relieve symptoms of gout.

HEADACHES AND MIGRAINES

Ginger: Ginger has been used for centuries to treat a variety of health conditions. Take ginger supplements or consume ginger tea or ginger powder to help relieve headache and migraine symptoms.

Peppermint Oil: Peppermint oil has a cooling and soothing effect on the head and neck. You can apply peppermint oil topically to the temples, neck, and forehead or inhale the scent of peppermint oil to help reduce headaches and migraines.

Feverfew is believed to help prevent the release of certain chemicals in the body that cause headaches and migraines. You can take feverfew supplements or consume feverfew tea to help reduce your risk of developing headaches and migraines.

Butterbur contains compounds that are believed to reduce inflammation and relax the blood vessels in the head, which can help to relieve headache pain. You can take butterbur supplements or drink butterbur tea to prevent headaches and migraines.

Magnesium is a mineral that helps to regulate muscle and nerve function, as well as the release of certain hormones in the body. Magnesium deficiencies have been linked to headaches and migraines, so increasing your intake of magnesium-rich foods, such as nuts, seeds, leafy greens, and whole grains, or taking magnesium supplements may help to reduce your symptoms.

HEARTBURN & INDIGESTION

Ginger contains compounds that can help reduce inflammation in the digestive tract and relieve symptoms of heartburn and indigestion. You can take ginger supplements or consume ginger tea or ginger powder to help relieve heartburn and indigestion.

Peppermint oil has been shown to have a calming effect on the digestive system. You can apply peppermint oil topically to the abdominal area or inhale the scent of peppermint oil to help reduce heartburn and indigestion.

Chamomile has been shown to have a relaxing effect on the digestive system. You can drink chamomile tea or take chamomile supplements to help relieve your symptoms.

Fennel has been shown to have antispasmodic properties, which can help to relieve symptoms of heartburn and indigestion by relaxing the muscles in the digestive tract. You can take fennel supplements or consume fennel tea or fennel seeds.

Licorice has been shown to have a soothing effect on the digestive system, which helps reduce symptoms of heartburn and indigestion. You can take licorice supplements or consume licorice tea.

HEMORRHOIDS

Hemorrhoids, also known as piles, are a common digestive issue that can cause discomfort and pain.

Witch hazel is a natural astringent that has been shown to reduce swelling and discomfort associated with hemorrhoids. You can apply witch hazel topically or use witch hazel wipes.

Aloe vera contains compounds that are believed to help reduce inflammation and soothe irritated skin, making it a great option for treating hemorrhoids. You can apply aloe vera gel topically or use aloe vera wipes to help reduce swelling and discomfort.

Horse chestnut contains compounds that are believed to help improve circulation and reduce swelling, making it an effective option for treating hemorrhoids. You can take horse chestnut supplements or apply horse chestnut cream topically.

Butcher's broom has been shown to have anti-inflammatory properties, which can help to reduce swelling and discomfort associated with hemorrhoids. You can take butcher's broom supplements or apply butcher's broom cream topically.

Calendula has been shown to have soothing properties, which can help to reduce irritation and discomfort associated with hemorrhoids. You can apply calendula cream topically to the affected area or use calendula wipes to help relieve your symptoms.

HIGH BLOOD PRESSURE / HYPERTENSION

High blood pressure, also known as hypertension, is a common condition that can increase the risk of heart disease, stroke, and other health problems.

Garlic contains compounds that have been shown to help lower blood pressure by relaxing blood vessels and improving blood flow. You can take garlic supplements or add garlic to your diet.

Coenzyme Q10 is an antioxidant that is found in many foods, including fatty fish, organ meats, and whole grains. You can also take CoQ10 supplements to help manage your blood pressure.

Celery seed contains compounds that are believed to help relax blood vessels, improve blood flow, and lower blood pressure. You can take celery seed supplements or add celery seed to your diet.

Hawthorn contains compounds that are believed to help relax blood vessels and improve blood flow, making it an effective option for managing high blood pressure. You can take hawthorn supplements or add hawthorn to your diet.

Magnesium helps to regulate the balance of fluids in the body and can help to relax blood vessels, which lowers blood pressure. You can take magnesium supplements or add magnesium-rich foods to your diet, such as leafy greens, nuts, and seeds.

HIGH CHOLESTEROL

High cholesterol is a common condition that can increase the risk of heart disease and stroke.

Oats are high in soluble fiber, which has been shown to help lower cholesterol levels by binding with cholesterol in the digestive system and removing it from the body. You can add oats to your diet by eating oatmeal for breakfast or adding oat bran to smoothies, baked goods, and other recipes.

Soluble fiber can also be found in other foods, such as beans, lentils, and apples, which can also help to lower cholesterol levels.

Garlic contains compounds that are believed to help reduce the amount of cholesterol produced by the liver and improve blood lipid levels. You can take garlic supplements or add garlic to your diet.

Red yeast rice contains compounds that are similar to those found in statin drugs, which are commonly used to treat high cholesterol. Take red yeast rice supplements or add red yeast rice to your diet.

Fish oil contains omega-3 fatty acids, which have been shown to help improve blood lipid levels and reduce the risk of heart disease. You can take fish oil supplements or add fish, such as salmon, to your diet to help improve your cholesterol levels.

INCONTINENCE

Incontinence, or the loss of bladder control, is a common condition that affects people of all ages. It can be an embarrassing and uncomfortable issue that can greatly impact a person's quality of life.

Pelvic floor exercises, also known as **Kegel exercises**, strengthen the muscles that control the bladder, reducing the frequency and severity of incontinence symptoms. To perform pelvic floor exercises, simply tighten the muscles you use to control urination, hold for a few seconds, and then release.

Dandelion root is a natural diuretic that can help to increase urine flow, reducing the frequency and severity of incontinence symptoms. You can take dandelion root supplements or add dandelion root tea to your daily routine.

Rooibos tea is believed to help reduce bladder muscle contractions and improve bladder control. You can drink rooibos tea on its own or add it to your diet as a caffeine-free alternative to coffee or tea.

Marshmallow root contains compounds that are believed to help soothe and protect the bladder, reducing the frequency and severity of incontinence symptoms. You can take marshmallow root supplements or add marshmallow root tea to your daily routine.

INGROWN TOENAIL

Ingrown toenails are a common foot problem that can cause pain, swelling, and redness around the affected nail. This condition occurs when the nail grows into the surrounding skin, causing it to become infected and painful.

1. **Epsom Salt** is a naturally occurring mineral that has been used for centuries to treat a variety of ailments. Soaking your affected foot in a warm bath of Epsom salt and water can reduce swelling and pain caused by an ingrown toenail.

2. **Tea tree oil** is a natural antiseptic and antifungal oil that has been used for centuries to treat skin infections and other conditions. When applied directly to an ingrown toenail, tea tree oil can help reduce inflammation and prevent the spread of infection. To use tea tree oil, simply dilute a few drops in a carrier oil such as coconut or olive oil, and apply it directly to the affected area using a cotton swab.

3. **Aloe vera** has anti-inflammatory properties that can help soothe irritated skin and reduce pain caused by an ingrown toenail. To use aloe vera, simply break off a piece of the plant and squeeze the gel directly onto the affected area.

4. **Garlic:** When applied directly to an ingrown toenail, garlic can help reduce inflammation and prevent the spread of infection. To use garlic, simply crush a clove of garlic and apply it directly to the affected area, or mix it with a carrier oil such as coconut or olive oil.

5. **Turmeric** is a spice whose anti-inflammatory properties can help reduce swelling and pain caused by an ingrown toenail. Simply mix a small amount of the spice with water to create a paste, and apply it directly to the affected area.

INSOMNIA

Insomnia is a sleep disorder that affects millions of people worldwide. Symptoms of insomnia can include difficulty falling asleep, waking up frequently during the night, and feeling tired or groggy during the day.

Valerian root is believed to have a calming effect on the body, helping to promote a restful sleep. You can take valerian root supplements or add valerian root tea to your daily routine.

Chamomile has a natural sedative effect. You can drink chamomile tea, or add chamomile to your bath to help you relax and fall asleep.

Lavender has a calming aroma that can help to promote relaxation and sleep. You can add a few drops of lavender oil to your pillow or use lavender-scented candles or sprays to help you fall asleep.

Magnesium helps to regulate the body's sleep-wake cycle and can promote relaxation, making it easier to fall asleep. You can take magnesium supplements, or add magnesium-rich foods like nuts, seeds, and leafy greens to your diet to help with insomnia.

JOINT PAIN & ARTHRITIS

Joint pain and arthritis are common conditions that can cause discomfort and limit mobility.

Turmeric contains curcumin, an anti-inflammatory compound that can help to reduce pain and swelling in the joints. You can add turmeric to your diet or take turmeric supplements.

Ginger has anti-inflammatory properties and can reduce pain and swelling in the joints. You can add ginger to your diet by grating fresh ginger root into your cooking or by drinking ginger tea.

Boswellia contains anti-inflammatory compounds that can help to reduce pain and swelling in the joints. You can take boswellia supplements or apply boswellia oil topically to the affected joint.

Devil's claw is a plant native to Africa with anti-inflammatory compounds that can reduce pain and swelling in the joints. You can take devil's claw supplements or drink devil's claw tea.

KIDNEY STONES

Kidney stones are small, hard deposits that can form in the kidneys and cause significant pain and discomfort.

Lemon juice is high in citric acid, which can help to dissolve kidney stones and reduce pain and discomfort. Add lemon juice to water or tea and drink it regularly.

Basil has antilithogenic properties, which means it can help to prevent the formation of kidney stones. You can add basil to your diet by using it in cooking or by drinking basil tea.

Parsley is a diuretic, which means it can help to increase urine flow and flush out kidney stones. You can add parsley to your diet by using it in cooking or by drinking parsley tea.

Dandelion has diuretic properties and can help to increase urine flow and flush out kidney stones. You can add dandelion to your diet by drinking dandelion tea or taking dandelion supplements.

MOTION SICKNESS, VERTIGO AND DIZZINESS

Motion sickness, vertigo, and dizziness are conditions that can cause discomfort and limit daily activities.

Ginger has anti-inflammatory properties and can help to reduce nausea and vomiting. You can add ginger to your diet by grating fresh ginger root into your cooking or by drinking ginger tea.

Peppermint has antispasmodic properties and can help to reduce nausea and vomiting. You can add peppermint to your diet by using it in cooking or by drinking peppermint tea.

Lavender has relaxing properties and can help to reduce anxiety and stress. You can add lavender to your daily routine by using lavender essential oil in aromatherapy or by drinking lavender tea.

Chamomile has relaxing properties and can help to reduce anxiety and stress. You can add chamomile to your daily routine by drinking chamomile tea or by using chamomile essential oil in aromatherapy.

MENSTRUAL PAIN

Menstrual pain, also known as dysmenorrhea, is a common condition experienced by many women.

Ginger has anti-inflammatory properties and can help to reduce pain and cramping associated with menstrual pain. You can add ginger to your diet or drink ginger tea.

Chamomile has relaxing properties and can help to reduce anxiety and stress associated with menstrual pain. You can add chamomile to your daily routine by drinking chamomile tea or by using chamomile essential oil in aromatherapy.

Evening primrose oil contains gamma-linolenic acid (GLA), an essential fatty acid that can help to reduce inflammation and pain associated with menstrual pain. You can add evening primrose oil to your routine by taking supplements or using topically.

Cinnamon has anti-inflammatory properties and can help to reduce pain and cramping. You can add cinnamon to your diet by using it in cooking or by drinking cinnamon tea.

MUSCLE CRAMPS

Magnesium is involved in muscle contraction and relaxation, and a deficiency can lead to muscle cramps. You can up your magnesium intake by eating magnesium-rich foods such as almonds, leafy greens, and avocados, or by taking magnesium supplements.

Potassium is involved in muscle function and helps regulate fluid balance in the body. Increase your potassium intake by eating potassium-rich foods such as bananas, sweet potatoes, and spinach.

Mustard seeds contain a compound called allyl isothiocyanate, which can help to reduce muscle cramps. Use them in cooking or take mustard seed supplements.

Chamomile has relaxing properties and can help to reduce muscle tension and spasms. Take by drinking chamomile tea or by using chamomile essential oil in aromatherapy.

NAIL FUNGUS

Nail fungus is a common condition that can cause thick, yellow, or brittle nails.

Tea tree oil has antifungal properties and can help to kill the fungus that is causing the infection. You can use tea tree oil by mixing it with a carrier oil, such as olive oil, and applying it directly.

Garlic has antifungal properties and can help to kill the fungus that is causing the infection. You can add garlic to your diet by eating raw garlic cloves or by taking garlic supplements.

Oregano oil has antifungal and antibacterial properties and can help to kill the fungus that is causing the infection. You can use oregano oil by mixing it with a carrier oil, such as olive oil, and applying it directly to the affected nail.

Apple cider vinegar has antifungal properties and can help to kill the fungus that is causing the infection. You can use apple cider vinegar by soaking your affected nail in a solution of water and apple cider vinegar for 15 to 20 minutes a day.

NAUSEA & VOMITING

Nausea and vomiting are common symptoms that can be caused by a variety of factors, including motion sickness, food poisoning, and certain medications.

Ginger has anti-inflammatory properties and can help to soothe an upset stomach. You can use ginger by drinking ginger tea, eating raw ginger, or taking ginger supplements.

Peppermint has antispasmodic properties and can help to calm an upset stomach. You can use peppermint by drinking peppermint tea, inhaling peppermint essential oil, or taking peppermint supplements.

Lemon has a fresh and soothing scent that calms an upset stomach. Use lemon by drinking lemon water, inhaling lemon essential oil, or using a lemon-scented product, like a candle or lotion.

Acupuncture is a form of traditional Chinese medicine that involves the insertion of very thin needles into specific points on the body. Acupuncture has been shown to be effective in treating nausea and vomiting and can help to improve digestive function.

NERVE PAIN

Nerve pain, also known as neuropathic pain, is a chronic condition that can be caused by a variety of factors, including injury, disease, and certain medications.

Turmeric contains curcumin, a powerful anti-inflammatory compound that has been shown to help reduce pain and improve nerve function. Use turmeric by taking turmeric supplements, drinking turmeric tea, or adding turmeric to your cooking.

Cayenne pepper contains capsaicin, a compound that has been shown to help reduce pain and improve nerve function. Use cayenne pepper by taking capsaicin supplements, applying a capsaicin cream to the affected area, or adding cayenne pepper to your cooking.

Alpha-Lipoic Acid is an antioxidant that has been shown to help reduce inflammation and improve nerve function. Use Alpha-Lipoic Acid by taking supplements, or applying a cream to affected area.

Magnesium can help to reduce inflammation and improve nerve function. Use magnesium by taking magnesium supplements, or eating magnesium-rich foods, such as nuts, seeds, and leafy greens.

NOSEBLEED

Nosebleeds can be a frustrating and uncomfortable experience, but they are generally not serious and can often be treated at home with natural remedies.

One of the most effective natural remedies for treating nosebleeds is to simply apply gentle pressure to the affected nostril for about 5-10 minutes. This can help to stop the bleeding and reduce any discomfort.

Saline nasal sprays can help to moisturize the nasal passages and reduce dryness, which is a common cause of nosebleeds. Spray the saline solution into your nostrils as directed on the packaging.

Topical Vitamin C has been shown to help improve blood vessel strength and reduce bleeding. You can use topical Vitamin C by applying a Vitamin C serum or cream to the inside of your nostrils.

Goldenrod has natural astringent properties that can help to stop bleeding and reduce inflammation. You can use goldenrod by making a tea or tincture, or by using a goldenrod extract or oil.

Finally, staying hydrated is an important part of preventing and treating nosebleeds. Drinking plenty of water and avoiding alcohol and caffeine can help to reduce dryness and keep the nasal passages moist.

PLANTAR FASCIITIS

Plantar fasciitis is a common foot condition that causes pain and discomfort in the heel and sole of the foot.

Stretching exercises: Gentle stretching exercises can reduce tension in the plantar fascia and improve flexibility in the foot. Effective stretches include calf stretches, foot flexes, and arch stretches.

Ice therapy: Applying ice to the affected area for 15-20 minutes several times a day can help to reduce pain and swelling. You can wrap a bag of ice in a towel or use a cold pack.

Massage: Massaging the foot, especially the heel and sole, can help to improve circulation and reduce pain. You can use a foam roller or a tennis ball to gently massage the affected area.

Ginger has anti-inflammatory properties that can help to reduce pain and swelling in the foot. You can consume ginger by drinking ginger tea or taking ginger supplements.

Turmeric: Like ginger, turmeric has anti-inflammatory properties that can help to relieve pain and swelling. You can consume turmeric by adding it to your food or taking turmeric supplements.

Willow bark has natural pain-relieving properties that make it a popular remedy for plantar fasciitis. You can take willow bark supplements or use a willow bark extract.

Capsaicin is a natural substance found in chili peppers that has pain-relieving properties. You can apply capsaicin cream to the affected area or take capsaicin supplements.

Arnica: Arnica is a natural remedy that has been used for centuries to relieve pain and swelling. You can apply arnica oil or cream to the affected area, or take arnica supplements.

POISON IVY/OAK/SUMAC

Poison ivy, poison oak, and poison sumac are all common plants that contain an allergenic oil called urushiol that can cause a skin rash and itching when it comes into contact with human skin.

Oatmeal has been used for centuries as a natural remedy for skin irritations and rashes. Grind oats into a fine powder and add it to a bath or make an oatmeal paste to apply directly to the affected area.

Aloe vera can help to relieve itching and redness. Apply aloe vera gel directly to the affected area or drink aloe vera juice.

Calamine lotion has a cooling effect that can help to relieve itching and redness. Apply calamine lotion directly to the affected area.

Witch hazel has astringent and anti-inflammatory properties that can help to reduce swelling and redness. You can apply witch hazel directly to the affected area or use a witch hazel-based skin lotion.

Baking soda can help to relieve itching and redness. Mix baking soda with water to form a paste and apply directly to affected area.

Apple cider vinegar has astringent properties that can help to relieve itching and redness. You can mix equal parts water and apple cider vinegar and apply directly to affected area with a cotton ball.

Essential oils such as tea tree, lavender, and eucalyptus have anti-inflammatory and soothing properties. Dilute essential oils in a carrier oil and apply directly to the affected area.

PSORIASIS OR RASH, DERMATITIS (ITCHY SKIN)

Aloe vera has anti-inflammatory and moisturizing properties that can help to soothe the skin and reduce redness and itching. Apply aloe vera gel directly to the affected area or drink aloe vera juice.

Omega-3 fatty acids: Omega-3 fatty acids, found in fatty fish, flaxseed, and chia seeds, have anti-inflammatory properties that can help to reduce the symptoms of psoriasis.

Turmeric has anti-inflammatory properties that can reduce symptoms of psoriasis. Take turmeric supplements or add turmeric to your diet in the form of a spice.

Dead Sea mud has been shown to reduce inflammation and soothe the skin. Use Dead Sea mud as a face mask or add it to your bath.

Vitamin D has been shown to help reduce symptoms of psoriasis. Take vitamin D supplements or get adequate sun exposure.

Tea tree oil: Tea tree oil has antifungal and antiseptic properties that can soothe the skin and reduce itching and redness. Add a few drops of tea tree oil to a carrier oil and apply directly to affected area.

Neem oil has anti-inflammatory and antifungal properties that help to soothe the skin and reduce itching and redness. Add a few drops of neem oil to a carrier oil and apply directly to the affected area.

SHINGLES

Shingles, also known as herpes zoster, is a viral infection that affects the nerve fibers and skin. It is caused by the varicella-zoster virus, which is the same virus that causes chickenpox. Symptoms of shingles can include a painful rash, blisters, itching, and burning sensations.

Lavender oil has antiseptic and pain-relieving properties that can soothe the skin and reduce itching and burning sensations. Apply lavender oil directly to the affected area or add it to a warm bath.

Licorice root has antiviral and anti-inflammatory properties that can help to reduce inflammation and relieve pain. You can take licorice root supplements or make licorice root tea.

Echinacea has antiviral properties that can help to boost the immune system and reduce the severity of shingles symptoms. You can take echinacea supplements or make

Lemon balm has antiviral and pain-relieving properties that can help to reduce the severity of shingles symptoms. You can apply lemon balm directly to the affected area or make lemon balm tea.

Capsaicin is an extract from chili peppers that has pain-relieving properties. You can apply capsaicin cream directly to affected areas.

Aloe vera has anti-inflammatory and moisturizing properties that can soothe the skin and reduce itching and burning. Apply aloe vera gel directly to the affected area or drink aloe vera juice.

Vitamin C has antiviral properties that can boost the immune system and reduce the severity of shingles. Take supplements or eat foods high in vitamin C, such as oranges and bell peppers.

SINUSITIS

Sinusitis is a condition characterized by inflammation of the sinuses, which can lead to symptoms such as nasal congestion, headache, and facial pain

Steam therapy can clear out mucus and relieve sinus pressure. Use a humidifier or take a hot shower to get benefits of steam therapy.

Saline solution can clean out the sinuses and reduce inflammation. Use a neti pot to flush out the sinuses with saline solution.

Ginger has anti-inflammatory properties that can help to reduce inflammation and relieve pain. You can take ginger supplements or drink ginger tea to get the benefits of ginger.

Eucalyptus oil has antibacterial and decongestant properties that can help to clear out mucus and relieve sinus pressure. You can inhale eucalyptus oil through a diffuser or add it to a steam bath.

Peppermint oil has antiseptic and decongestant properties that can help to clear out mucus and relieve sinus pressure. You can inhale peppermint oil through a diffuser or add it to a steam bath.

Vitamin C has antioxidant properties that can help to reduce inflammation and boost the immune system. Take supplements or eat foods high in vitamin C, such as oranges and bell peppers.

Probiotics can help to boost the immune system and reduce inflammation. You can take probiotic supplements or eat foods high in probiotics, such as yogurt and kefir.

SKIN FUNGUS

Skin fungus is a common condition that can cause symptoms such as itching, redness, and scaling.

Tea tree oil has antifungal and antiseptic properties that can help to kill the fungus and promote healing. Apply tea tree oil directly to the affected area or add it to a carrier oil, such as coconut oil.

Garlic has antifungal properties that can help to kill the fungus and reduce inflammation. You can apply crushed garlic directly to the affected area or take garlic supplements.

Aloe vera has antibacterial and anti-inflammatory properties that can help to soothe the skin and reduce redness. You can apply aloe vera gel directly to the affected area.

Apple cider vinegar has antifungal and antibacterial properties that can help to kill the fungus and promote healing. You can dilute apple cider vinegar with water and apply it directly to affected area.

Oregano oil has antifungal and antiseptic properties that can help to kill the fungus and promote healing. You can apply oregano oil directly to the affected area or take oregano oil supplements.

Coconut oil has antifungal and antibacterial properties that help to kill the fungus and promote healing. Apply directly to affected area.

Vitamin E has antioxidant and anti-inflammatory properties that can help to soothe the skin and reduce redness. Apply vitamin E oil directly to the affected area or take vitamin E supplements.

SPLINTERS

Salt water can help to reduce swelling and clean the area around the splinter. Mix a pinch of salt with warm water and soak the affected area for 10-15 minutes.

Honey has antibacterial and anti-inflammatory properties that can help to soothe the skin and reduce swelling. You can apply honey directly to the affected area and cover with a bandage.

Aloe vera has antibacterial and anti-inflammatory properties that can help to soothe the skin and reduce swelling. You can apply aloe vera gel directly to the affected area.

Tea tree oil has antiseptic and antimicrobial properties that can help to prevent infection and promote healing. Apply tea tree oil directly to the affected area or add it to a carrier oil, such as coconut oil.

Echinacea is a herb that has immune-boosting properties that can help to prevent infection and promote healing. Take echinacea supplements or apply echinacea tincture directly to the affected area.

Lavender oil has antiseptic and anti-inflammatory properties that can help to soothe the skin and reduce swelling. Apply lavender oil directly to affected area or add it to a carrier oil, such as coconut oil.

Turmeric is a spice that has anti-inflammatory properties that can help to reduce swelling and promote healing. Apply turmeric paste directly to the affected area or take turmeric supplements.

STINKY FEET

Stinky feet can be an embarrassing and unpleasant problem, but it is a common one. The odor is often caused by bacteria and fungi that thrive in warm and moist environments, such as shoes and socks.

Tea tree oil: This essential oil has antimicrobial properties and can help kill the bacteria and fungi that cause odor. Mix a few drops of tea tree oil with coconut oil or olive oil and massage into your feet.

Apple cider vinegar: This natural astringent can help neutralize odor and balance the pH level of your skin. Mix equal parts of apple cider vinegar and water in a spray bottle, and spritz your feet after showering. Let dry completely before putting on socks and shoes.

Baking soda: This natural deodorizer can help absorb the odor-causing bacteria on your feet. Mix baking soda with water to form a paste and apply it to your feet. Leave it on for a few minutes, then rinse with water.

Sage: This herb has antifungal properties and can help eliminate foot odor. Boil 1 cup of sage in 2 cups of water for 15 minutes, then strain. Soak your feet in the warm tea for 20-30 minutes.

Chamomile: This herb has antiseptic and anti-inflammatory properties. Boil 2-3 chamomile tea bags in 1 cup of water for 10 minutes, then strain. Soak feet in the warm tea for 15-20 minutes.

Cornstarch: This natural absorbent can help absorb sweat and neutralize foot odor. Sprinkle some cornstarch into your shoes or socks, or directly onto your feet, to help keep them dry and fresh.

STREP THROAT

Strep throat is a common illness that can cause severe pain and discomfort in the throat. It is caused by a bacterial infection, and it often requires antibiotics to fully treat it.

Salt Water Gargle: Gargling salt water several times a day can help reduce pain and swelling in the throat. Mix a quarter teaspoon of salt into a glass of warm water and gargle for about 30 seconds.

Honey has natural antibacterial properties, and it can help soothe the throat and reduce pain. Simply stir a spoonful of honey into a cup of warm water or tea, and drink it several times a day.

Lemon has antibacterial and anti-inflammatory properties, making it a great natural remedy. Squeeze fresh lemon juice into a glass of warm water and add a spoonful of honey for a soothing lemon tea.

Ginger can help reduce pain and inflammation in the throat. Boil slices of fresh ginger in water to make a tea, or add fresh grated ginger to a glass of warm water and drink it several times a day.

Garlic is another natural remedy with strong antibacterial properties. Crush fresh garlic cloves and add them to warm water or tea, or simply eat raw garlic cloves several times a day.

Echinacea can be used to boost the immune system and fight infections. Echinacea supplements or tea can be taken several times a day to help reduce the symptoms of strep throat.

SUNBURN

Sunburns are a common skin condition that occurs when skin is exposed to harmful ultraviolet (UV) rays from the sun. It can cause red, painful, and peeling skin that can last for several days.

Aloe Vera is a popular natural remedy for sunburns due to its moisturizing and anti-inflammatory properties. Its gel can be applied directly to sunburned skin for a soothing effect.

Oatmeal has anti-inflammatory properties that can help to reduce pain and itching, and its moisturizing properties can help to hydrate and heal sunburned skin. To use oatmeal for sunburns, simply add a cup of oats to a bathtub of cool water and soak for 15 to 20 minutes.

Green tea contains antioxidants and anti-inflammatory properties that can help to reduce pain and inflammation caused by sunburns. To use green tea for sunburns, simply soak a few green tea bags in cool water and apply the tea to sunburned skin using a cloth.

Vinegar can help to soothe sunburned skin and reduce pain and itching. To use vinegar for sunburns, mix equal parts of vinegar and water and apply the mixture to sunburned skin using a cloth.

Coconut oil is a natural moisturizer that can soothe sunburned skin and reduce pain and itching. Its antioxidants can also help to heal damaged skin. Apply coconut oil directly to sunburned skin.

Calendula has anti-inflammatory properties that can help to reduce pain and inflammation, while its antioxidants can help to heal damaged skin. Calendula can be found in the form of creams, gels, and lotions that can be applied directly to sunburned skin.

Lavender is another herb that has been used for centuries to treat skin conditions, including sunburns. Its anti-inflammatory properties can help to soothe sunburned skin and reduce pain and itching.

TINNITUS

Tinnitus is a condition characterized by ringing or buzzing in the ears, and it affects millions of people worldwide.

Ginkgo Biloba has been shown to be effective in reducing tinnitus symptoms and improving overall hearing health. Ginkgo Biloba is available in supplement form and can be taken orally.

Magnesium has been shown to be effective in reducing tinnitus symptoms and improving overall hearing health. Magnesium is available in supplement form and can be taken orally.

Zinc has been shown to be effective in reducing tinnitus symptoms and improving overall hearing health. Zinc is available in supplement form and can be taken orally.

B vitamins, particularly B12 and folate, have been shown to be effective in reducing tinnitus symptoms and improving overall hearing health. B vitamins are also available in supplement form.

Omega-3 fatty acids have been shown to be effective in reducing tinnitus symptoms and improving overall hearing health. Omega-3 fatty acids are available in supplement form and can be taken orally.

Herbs such as ginseng, garlic, and hawthorn have also been shown to be effective in reducing tinnitus symptoms and improving overall hearing health.

TOOTHACHES

Toothaches can be one of the most painful and disruptive experiences one can go through. The throbbing pain can make it difficult to sleep, eat, or even speak.

Cloves have been used for centuries to treat toothaches. The oil from the clove contains eugenol, which has both antiseptic and anesthetic properties. To use cloves for a toothache, simply place a whole clove on the affected area, or mix clove oil with a carrier oil and use a cotton ball to apply it directly to the tooth.

Saltwater Rinse: Saltwater can help relieve pain and reduce inflammation in the mouth. To use, mix one teaspoon of salt into a glass of warm water, and rinse your mouth with the solution for 30 seconds. Repeat as necessary.

Garlic has both antibacterial and pain-relieving properties, making it an excellent natural remedy for toothaches. Simply chew on a clove of garlic or crush it and apply it directly to the affected area.

Peppermint oil contains menthol, which has a cooling and numbing effect on the skin and can help alleviate toothache pain. To use, mix a few drops of peppermint oil with a carrier oil, such as coconut oil, and apply it to the affected area using a cotton ball.

Ginger is a natural anti-inflammatory, making it a great option for reducing swelling and pain. Simply chew on a piece of fresh ginger root or make a tea by steeping sliced ginger in hot water.

Willow bark contains salicin, which is a natural pain reliever and anti-inflammatory. To use, steep willow bark in hot water to make a tea, or take it in supplement form.

WARTS

Warts are small growths that can appear on the skin and are caused by a virus known as the human papillomavirus (HPV). While warts are generally harmless, they can be unsightly and uncomfortable.

Apple cider vinegar is a popular natural remedy for warts due to its acidic properties. Soak a cotton ball in apple cider vinegar and apply it to the wart, securing it in place with a bandage. Repeat several times a day for several weeks until the wart disappears.

Garlic has antimicrobial and antiviral properties, making it an effective natural remedy for warts. Crush a clove of garlic and apply it directly to the wart, securing it in place with a bandage. Repeat several times a day for several weeks until the wart disappears.

Dandelion sap is a natural remedy for warts that has been used for centuries. To use, simply break the stem of a dandelion plant and allow the sap to flow over the wart. Repeat this process several times a day for several weeks until the wart disappears.

Tree oil is a natural antiseptic and has been shown to be effective in treating warts. Dilute tea tree oil with a carrier oil, such as coconut oil, and apply it directly to the wart using a cotton ball. Repeat several times a day for several weeks until the wart disappears.

Vitamin C is an antioxidant that can boost the immune system and fight the virus that causes warts. Take vitamin C supplements or eat foods such as oranges, strawberries, and bell peppers.

Aloe vera is a natural moisturizer and has antiviral properties, making it an effective natural remedy for warts. Break off a piece of an aloe vera plant and apply the gel directly to the wart. Repeat this process several times a day until the wart disappears.

WOUNDS

Wounds can range from minor cuts and scrapes to more serious injuries, and proper wound care is essential to prevent infection and promote healing.

Honey has antimicrobial properties and can help prevent infection in wounds. It also promotes healing by keeping the wound moist and reducing inflammation. To use, simply apply honey directly to the wound and cover it with a bandage.

Aloe vera is a natural moisturizer and has anti-inflammatory properties, making it an effective remedy for wounds. Break off a piece of an aloe vera plant and apply the gel directly to the wound.

Turmeric is a powerful anti-inflammatory herb that can help prevent infection in wounds. To use, make a paste using turmeric powder and water, and apply it directly to the wound.

Calendula is an herb that has antimicrobial and anti-inflammatory properties, making it an effective natural remedy for wounds. To use, make a calendula ointment by mixing dried calendula flowers with olive oil and beeswax, and apply it directly to the wound.

Witch hazel is a natural astringent and has anti-inflammatory properties, making it an effective natural remedy for wounds. Simply apply witch hazel directly to the wound using a cotton ball.

Tea tree oil is a natural antiseptic effective in treating wounds. To use, dilute tea tree oil with a carrier oil, such as coconut oil, and apply it directly to the wound using a cotton ball.

WEIRD FORGOTTEN REMEDIES

TREATING YOUR PAIN THE NATURAL WAY

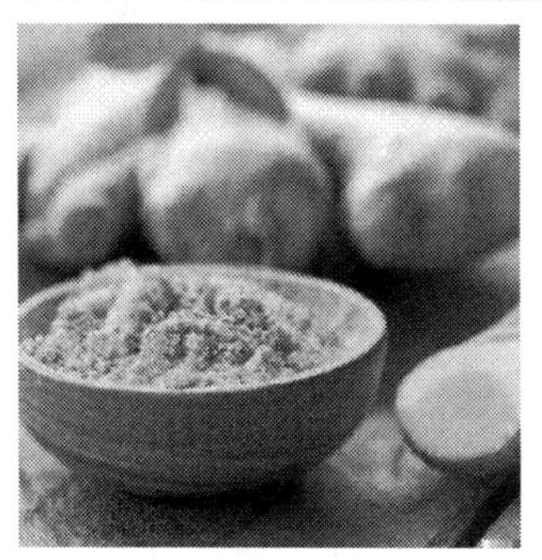

You may look to natural supplements and herbs as alternatives to traditional pain relievers and opioids. Here are a few of the most commonly used natural supplements and herbs for pain relief:

Turmeric has anti-inflammatory and pain-relieving properties. The active ingredient in turmeric, curcumin, has been shown to reduce pain and improve mobility in people with joint pain.

Devil's claw root is a plant that is native to Africa and is used in traditional medicine to relieve pain and inflammation. It is commonly used to relieve back pain, arthritis pain, and headaches.

Capsaicin works by reducing the levels of substance P, a chemical in the body that contributes to pain perception. Capsaicin is available in creams, gels, and patches, and can be applied topically to relieve pain in the joints, muscles, and skin.

Comfrey has anti-inflammatory and pain-relieving properties. Comfrey is commonly used to relieve pain in the joints and muscles.

Glucosamine supplements have been shown to relieve pain and improve joint function in people with osteoarthritis.

Boswellia is used in traditional medicine to relieve pain and inflammation. Boswellia contains compounds that have anti-inflammatory and pain-relieving properties.

COULD THIS NATURAL PAIN KILLER BE GROWING IN YOUR BACKYARD?

Wild lettuce, also known as Lactuca virosa, is a common weed that grows in many parts of the world. Despite its humble appearance, wild lettuce has been used for centuries as an all-natural pain reliever. It is considered a safe and effective alternative to over-the-counter pain medications for many types of pain, including headache, menstrual cramps, muscle pain, and joint pain.

Identifying Wild Lettuce:

Wild lettuce is a tall, leafy plant that can grow up to six feet in height. It has narrow leaves that are green on top and white on the bottom. The plant produces small, yellow flowers and has a milky sap that is produced when the stem is broken or the leaves are torn. Wild lettuce can be found growing in fields, along roadsides, and in other areas where the soil is disturbed.

Growing Wild Lettuce:

Wild lettuce is easy to grow and can be started from seed. It can be grown in a garden, or in pots if space is limited. The plant prefers full sun and well-drained soil. It is also relatively drought-tolerant, and does not require frequent watering. Once established, wild lettuce will grow rapidly and will produce new leaves and flowers throughout the growing season.

Using Wild Lettuce for Pain Relief:

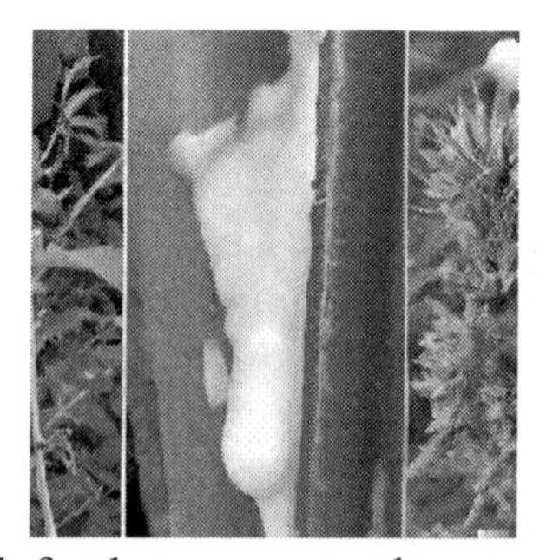

Wild lettuce is most used as a sedative and pain reliever. The milky sap from the plant contains compounds that have a relaxing effect on the body, helping to reduce pain and tension.

Wild lettuce can be ingested as a tea, tincture, or capsule. To make a tea, simply steep a few leaves in hot water for several minutes. Tinctures can be purchased at health food stores or can be made at home by soaking the leaves in alcohol or vinegar. Capsules are also available, and can be found at many health food stores or online.

It is important to note that wild lettuce should be used with caution, as it can have mild side effects such as drowsiness or upset stomach. If you are pregnant or nursing, it is best to avoid using wild lettuce, as its effects on pregnancy and lactation are not well understood.

USE THIS DIY ANTIBIOTIC OINTMENT TO TREAT WOUNDS

Antibiotic ointments are a common treatment for various skin conditions, such as cuts, scrapes, and minor infections.

Ingredients:

- 1/4 cup of beeswax
- 1/2 cup of coconut oil
- 1/4 cup of olive oil
- 10 drops of tea tree essential oil
- 10 drops of lavender essential oil

Instructions:

1. Combine the beeswax, coconut oil, and olive oil in a double boiler or a heat-proof bowl over a pot of simmering water. Stir the ingredients until they are fully melted.
2. Remove the double boiler or heat-proof bowl from the heat and let it cool for a few minutes.
3. Add the tea tree and lavender essential oils to the melted mixture and stir well.
4. Pour the mixture into a sterilized glass jar and let it cool completely.
5. Once the ointment has cooled, close the jar and label it with the date and ingredients.

Your homemade antibiotic ointment is now ready to use! The beeswax and coconut oil will help create a protective barrier on the skin, while the olive oil and essential oils will provide antibacterial and anti-inflammatory benefits.

WHY YOU SHOULD CONSIDER SLEEPING WITH AN ONION IN YOUR SOCK

If you're looking for a natural, simple way to improve your health, you might want to consider slipping an onion in your sock before you go to bed. This may sound strange, but it's a traditional remedy that has been passed down for generations and is said to provide a range of health benefits.

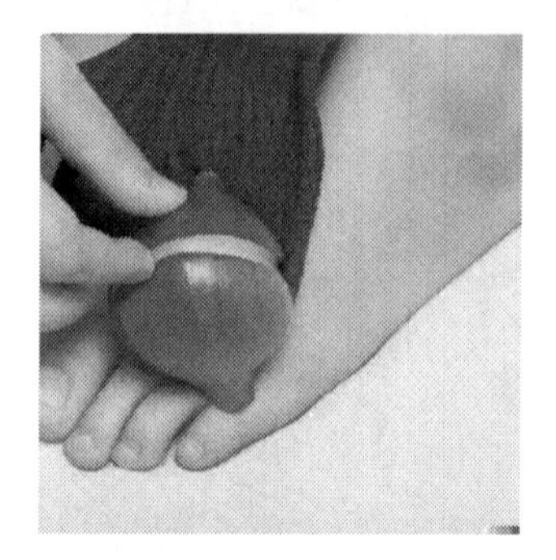

The origins of the onion-in-the-sock remedy are unclear, but it's believed to have been used by people for centuries to improve their health and well-being. The idea is that you place a sliced onion in your sock before going to bed and leave it there overnight. As you sleep, the onion is said to release its healing properties into your body, providing you with a range of health benefits.

Immune Boosting: Onions contain a range of antioxidants and anti-inflammatory compounds that are known to help strengthen the immune system and protect against illness. By sleeping with an onion in your sock, you're said to be able to absorb these compounds into your body, helping to keep you healthy and protected from illness.

Improved Circulation: Onions contain compounds that can help to increase blood flow and reduce inflammation in the body. By sleeping with an onion in your sock, you're said to be able to improve the circulation in your feet, which can help to reduce swelling, discomfort, and pain.

Skin Health: Onions contain compounds that help cleanse the skin and reduce inflammation, which can help improve the appearance of your skin and prevent skin problems like acne and eczema.

WHY YOU SHOULD PUT GARLIC IN YOUR EAR BEFORE GOING TO BED

While it's often used to add flavor to dishes, it may also have a surprising use before bedtime: putting garlic in your ear. This may sound unusual, but it's a practice that has been used for centuries to treat various health conditions, including ear infections, ear pain, and ringing in the ears (tinnitus).

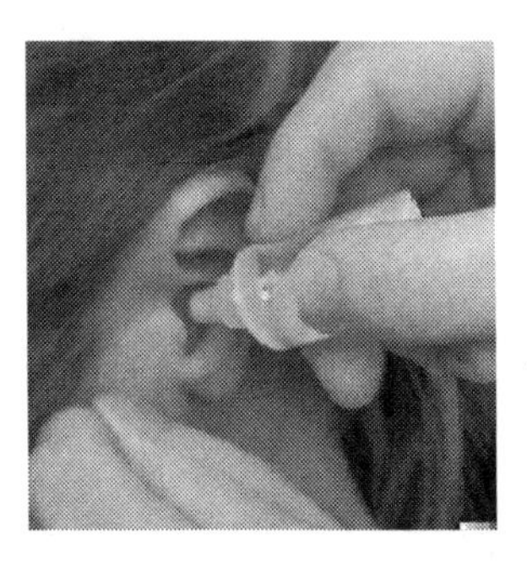

First, let's look at the benefits of garlic for ear infections. Garlic is a natural antiseptic and has antibacterial properties, making it an effective treatment for ear infections. When put into the ear, the juice from crushed garlic can help fight off the bacteria that cause ear infections, reducing inflammation and relieving pain.

Garlic can also help relieve ear pain, often caused by ear infections. The anti-inflammatory properties of garlic can help reduce swelling and discomfort in the ear, making it easier to fall asleep.

In addition to its benefits for ear infections and ear pain, garlic can also help treat ringing in the ears (tinnitus). Tinnitus is often caused by inflammation in the ear, and the anti-inflammatory properties of garlic can help reduce ringing in the ears.

To do this, simply crush a clove of garlic and extract the juice. Next, soak a cotton ball in the garlic juice and place it in your ear, leaving it in overnight. This can help treat ear infections, relieve ear pain, and reduce ringing in the ears.

THE AMAZING INFLAMMATION BUSTING POWER OF CABBAGE WRAPS

Joint pain and swelling can be incredibly debilitating and can make even the simplest tasks difficult. One amazing remedy to alleviate these problems is the cabbage leaf wrap.

What you'll need:

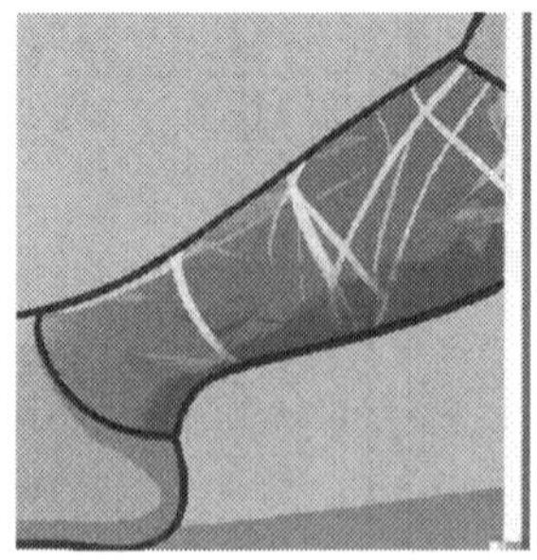

- 1 large cabbage leaf
- A microwave or a saucepan
- A towel
- Tape or a bandage

Instructions:

1. Remove a large cabbage leaf from the head of a cabbage. Rinse the leaf to remove any dirt or debris.
2. If you're using a microwave, place the leaf in the microwave for 30-45 seconds, or until it is soft and pliable. If you're using a saucepan, bring a pot of water to a boil and place the leaf in the boiling water for 1-2 minutes, or until it is soft and pliable.
3. Carefully remove the leaf from the microwave or saucepan and place it on a towel. Allow it to cool for a minute or two, until it is comfortable to the touch.
4. Place the leaf on the affected joint, with the inside of the leaf facing the skin. Wrap the leaf around the joint, securing it with tape or a bandage.
5. Leave the wrap in place for 30 minutes to an hour. If the wrap starts to feel too warm, remove it and place it in the refrigerator for a few minutes before re-applying.

Why it works: Cabbage leaves contain several anti-inflammatory compounds that help to reduce swelling and pain. When the cabbage leaf is heated, these compounds are released, making them more easily absorbed into the skin. The warmth also helps increase blood flow to the affected area, helping to reduce pain and swelling.

The cabbage leaf wrap also has a cooling effect, helping to reduce inflammation and provide relief from joint pain. This makes it an ideal remedy for arthritis, tendonitis, and bursitis.

HOW TO MAKE YOUR OWN CALCIUM PILL SUPPLEMENTS AT HOME FROM EGGSHELLS!

Calcium is an essential mineral that is important for maintaining strong bones and teeth, as well as for supporting a healthy cardiovascular system. Here's a forgotten skill our grandparents used to make their own bone strengthening calcium pills or powder.

What you'll need:

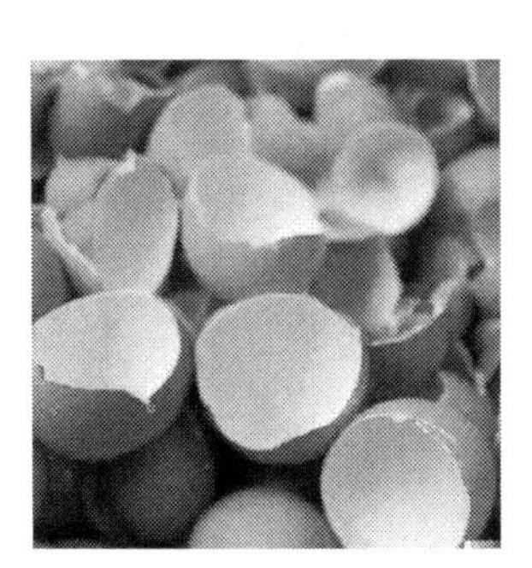

- 12 eggshells
- A baking sheet
- A coffee grinder or a mortar and pestle
- A strainer or cheesecloth
- A bowl
- Gelatin or empty gelatin capsules

Instructions:

1. Rinse the eggshells and let them dry completely. This will help to remove any bacteria or other contaminants.
2. Once the eggshells are dry, place them on a baking sheet and bake them in the oven at 300°F for 10-15 minutes. This will help to remove any remaining bacteria and make the eggshells easier to grind.
3. Remove the eggshells from the oven and let them cool completely.
4. Grind the eggshells into a fine powder using a coffee grinder or a mortar and pestle.
5. Strain the eggshell powder through a strainer or cheesecloth to remove any larger pieces.
6. Pour the eggshell powder into a bowl and add enough water to make a paste. Stir the paste until it is smooth.
7. Fill empty gelatin capsules with the eggshell paste or mix the paste with gelatin to make calcium pills.

Why it works: Eggshells are a rich source of calcium carbonate, which is the same form of calcium found in many store-bought calcium supplements.

HOW TO USE SALT AND OIL FOR TOOTH AND GUM DECAY WHEN YOU CAN'T GET TO THE DENTIST

Tooth and gum decay is a common problem that can cause pain, sensitivity, and other oral health issues. One often ignored remedy is the salt and oil rinse, which is a simple and effective way to improve oral health and reduce the risk of decay.

What you'll need:

- 1 teaspoon of salt
- 1 tablespoon of oil (such as olive, coconut, or sesame oil)
- A cup
- Warm water

Instructions:

1. Combine the salt and oil in a cup. Stir until the salt is fully dissolved.
2. Add warm water to the cup and stir to combine.
3. Rinse your mouth with the salt and oil solution for 2-3 minutes, making sure to swish the solution around all parts of your mouth, including your teeth and gums.
4. Spit out the solution and rinse your mouth with warm water.
5. Repeat the salt and oil rinse once or twice a week, or as needed.

Why it works: Salt has antiseptic properties that can help to kill bacteria and reduce the risk of decay. Salt can also help to reduce inflammation and promote healing, making it an effective treatment for gum disease.

Oil, on the other hand, has antibacterial properties that can help to remove plaque and other debris from the teeth and gums. It can also help to reduce inflammation and promote healing, making it an effective treatment for gum disease.

Salt and oil can provide a powerful and effective treatment for tooth and gum decay. This makes the salt and oil rinse an effective and natural alternative to traditional oral care products.

DON'T THROW AWAY YOUR ONION SKINS! DO THIS INSTEAD...

Onion skins are a treasure trove of health benefits and medicinal uses. From boosting the immune system to relieving pain, they have a wide range of benefits and are a must-have in your pantry.

1. **Boosts the Immune System**: Onion skins are rich in antioxidants, like quercetin, which has been shown to boost the immune system and protect against illnesses. Make a tea by simmering the skins in water for about 10 minutes then straining the liquid. Drink daily to boost immune system.
2. **Pain Relief**: Onion skins contain anti-inflammatory compounds that can help relieve pain, particularly in the joints. Make a poultice by boiling the skins in water, straining the liquid, then soaking a cloth in the liquid. Apply the cloth to the affected area for 20-30 minutes.
3. **Promotes Healthy Skin**: Onion skins contain sulfur, an important mineral for healthy skin. Make a face mask by grinding the skins into a fine powder and mixing it with water to form a paste. Apply paste to your face and leave it on for 15-20 minutes before rinsing it off with warm water.
4. **Supports Digestive Health**: Onion skins contain fiber, which is important for digestive health. Add to soups and stews or use to make a tea. This will keep your digestive system running smoothly and prevent constipation.
5. **Reduces Inflammation**: Onion skins contain anti-inflammatory compounds that can help reduce inflammation in the body. Make a tea by simmering the skins in water for

about 10 minutes and then straining the liquid. Drink this tea daily to reduce inflammation.

DRINK A CUP OF THIS WEIRD LIQUID EACH NIGHT TO SLEEP LIKE A BABY!

Kefir is a fermented milk drink that has numerous health benefits. One of the benefits of kefir is its ability to help you sleep better. If you're having trouble sleeping, kefir might just be the answer.

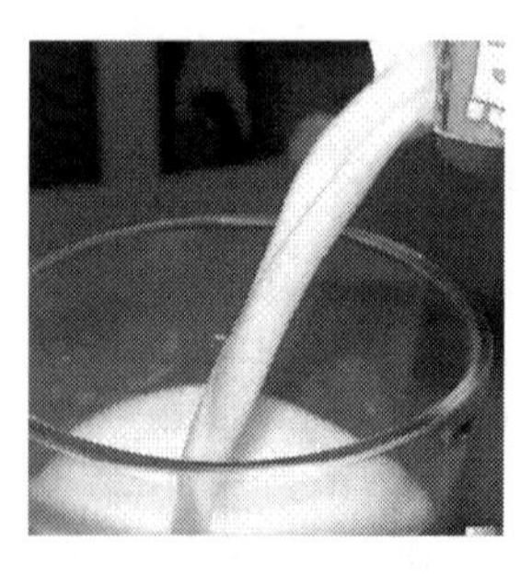

Kefir is rich in probiotics, which are beneficial bacteria that can improve our gut health and have been found to have a positive impact on our sleep, as they help regulate the production of hormones that control our sleep-wake cycle. Additionally, the probiotics in kefir can help improve our immune system, which can make us feel more relaxed and calmer, improving our sleep quality.

Kefir is also a good source of calcium, which is important for good sleep and helps regulate the production of melatonin, a hormone that regulates our sleep-wake cycle. Consuming kefir can ensure that your body has enough calcium to produce the right amount of melatonin, helping you fall asleep faster and longer.

Another way kefir can improve sleep is by reducing inflammation. Inflammation is a common cause of sleep problems, as it can cause discomfort and pain that makes it difficult to fall asleep and stay asleep. Kefir contains anti-inflammatory properties that can help reduce inflammation in the body. Experts recommend consuming around 8 ounces of kefir per day to see the best results.

YOUR MEDICINAL HERB GARDEN: PLANT THESE 16 HERBS

ECHINACEA

Echinacea, also known as the purple coneflower, is a medicinal herb widely used for its natural immune-boosting properties. Growing echinacea in a medicinal herb garden is an excellent way to have a readily available source of this versatile plant.

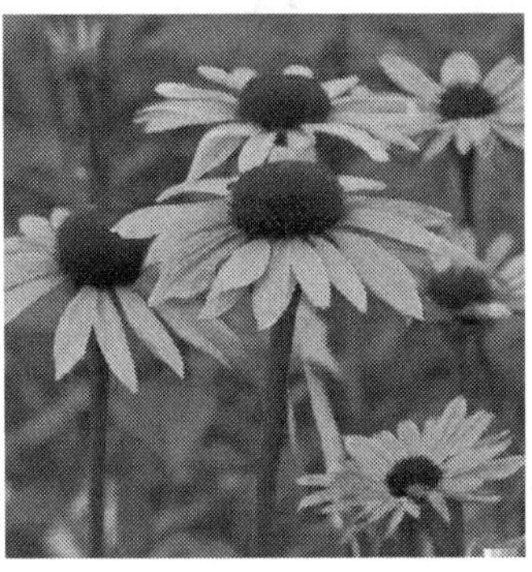

To grow echinacea, it is best to plant the seeds in the spring or fall. Choose a location in your garden that gets plenty of sunlight, as echinacea prefers full sun to partial shade. Prepare the soil before planting by adding compost or well-rotted manure to improve its fertility. Space the seeds or plants out a few feet apart to allow for adequate air flow and to prevent the growth of any fungal diseases.

Echinacea is known for its ability to support the immune system, making it an excellent herb for the colder months. Its antiviral and antibacterial properties make it a great choice for preventing and treating infections, including colds and the flu. It can also be used topically to treat skin infections and wounds, and it is often used as a remedy for sore throat, sinusitis, and other respiratory conditions.

While echinacea is generally considered to be safe, it is important to note that some people may experience side effects when using this herb. These can include allergic reactions, digestive upset, and increased sensitivity to sunlight. If you are taking any prescription medications, it is always best to talk to your healthcare provider before using echinacea, as it may interact with certain drugs.

CALENDULA, POT MARIGOLD

Calendula, also known as pot marigold, is a bright and cheerful herb that has been used for centuries for its medicinal properties. This easy-to-grow annual is a great addition to any medicinal herb garden, and it can be used for a variety of health conditions.

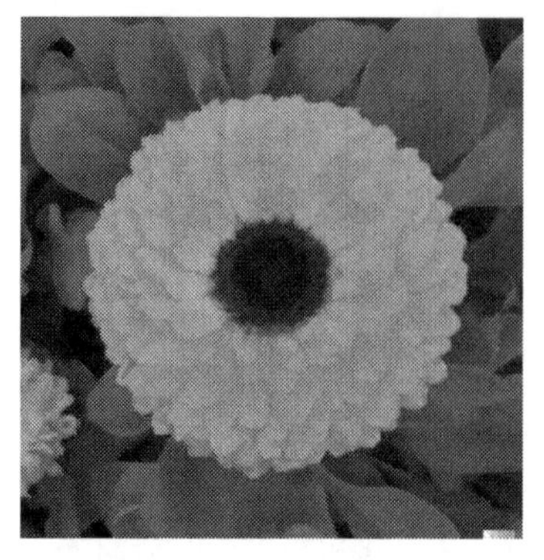

To grow calendula, choose a location in your garden that receives full sun to partial shade. The soil should be well-drained prepared by adding compost or well-rotted manure to improve its fertility. Calendula can be planted from seed directly in the spring outdoors, or you can start it indoors a few weeks before the last frost date.

Calendula is known for its anti-inflammatory, antiseptic, and wound-healing properties. It is often used topically to soothe skin irritations, burns, or cuts. It is also used for digestive problems, menstrual cramps, or respiratory infections. The flowers can be made into a tea, tincture, or ointment and applied directly to skin.

While calendula is generally considered to be safe, it is important to note that some people may experience allergic reactions when using this herb. If you have an allergy to plants in the daisy family, it is best to avoid using calendula. Also, it is always best to talk to your healthcare provider before using any herbal remedies, especially if you are pregnant, breastfeeding, or taking prescription medications.

MOTHERWORT

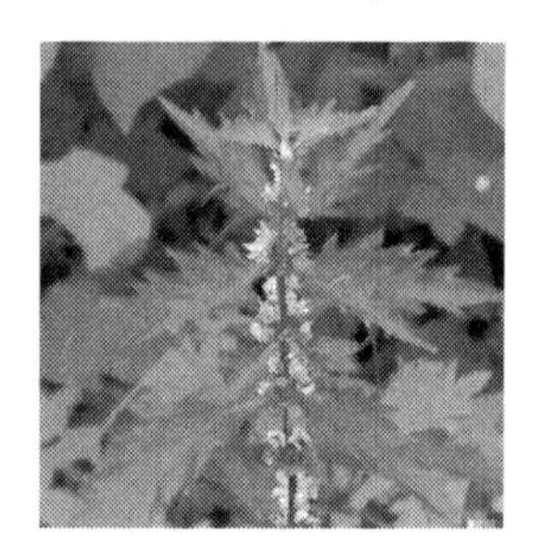

Motherwort (Leonurus cardiaca) is a robust, hardy herb known for its medicinal properties. It is native to Europe and Asia, but has naturalized in many parts of the world and can be found growing wild in many regions. Motherwort is a popular herb to grow in a medicinal herb garden due to its versatility and effectiveness.

To grow motherwort, choose a location in your garden that receives full sun to partial shade. The soil should be well-drained and rich in organic matter, and you may need to amend it with compost or well-rotted manure to improve its fertility. It can be propagated from seed, division, or cuttings, and it is best planted in the spring.

Motherwort has a long history of use as a medicinal herb, and it is especially well known for its calming and heart-nourishing properties. It is used to soothe anxiety, heart palpitations, and high blood pressure. It is also used to support women during menopause, menstruation, and childbirth. The leaves and flowers can be made into a tea, tincture, or ointment, and it is often used in combination with other herbs for maximum effectiveness.

While motherwort is generally considered to be safe, it is important to note that it can interact with some prescription medications, including blood thinners, beta-blockers, and calcium channel blockers.

PASSIONFLOWER

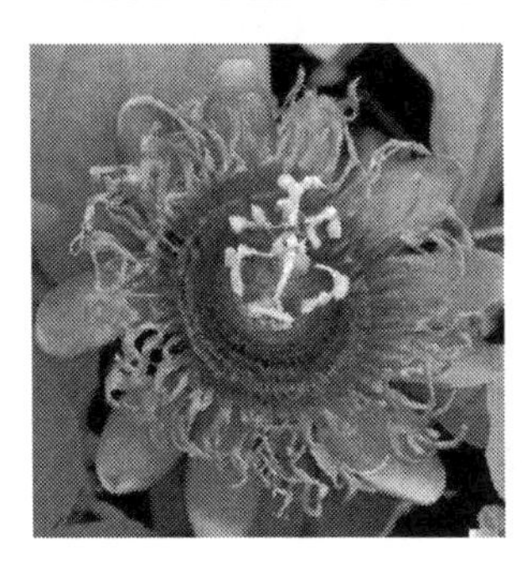

Passionflower (Passiflora incarnata) is a beautiful and fragrant herb that is prized for its medicinal properties. This climbing vine is native to the Americas, but it can now be found growing in many parts of the world. Passionflower is a popular herb to grow in a medicinal herb garden due to its effectiveness in treating a variety of conditions, including anxiety, insomnia, and pain.

To grow passionflower, you will need to choose a location in your garden that provides full sun to partial shade. The soil should be well-drained and rich in organic matter, and you may need to amend it with compost or well-rotted manure to improve its fertility.

Passionflower can be propagated from seed, division, or cuttings, and it is best planted in the spring.

Passionflower is used for its calming and pain-relieving properties, and it is often used to treat anxiety, insomnia, and pain associated with conditions like headaches, muscle cramps, and menstrual cramps. The leaves, stems, and flowers can be made into a tea, tincture, or ointment, and it is often used in combination with other herbs for maximum effectiveness.

While passionflower is generally considered to be safe, it is important to note that it can interact with some prescription medications, including sedatives, benzodiazepines, and anti-anxiety medications.

HOLY BASIL

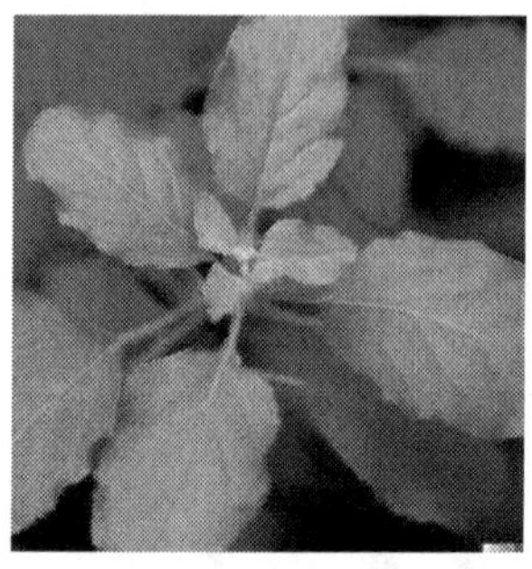

Holy basil (Ocimum sanctum), also known as Tulsi, is a fragrant herb that is widely used in Ayurvedic medicine for its health-promoting properties. This herb is native to India and Southeast Asia, but it can now be found growing in many parts of the world. Holy basil is a popular herb to grow in a medicinal herb garden, and it is prized for its ability to support the immune system, promote healthy digestion, and reduce stress and anxiety.

To grow holy basil, you will need to choose a location in your garden that provides full sun to partial shade. The soil should be well-drained and rich in organic matter, and you may need to amend it with compost or well-rotted manure to improve its fertility. Holy basil can be propagated from seed, division, or cuttings, and it is best planted in the spring.

Holy basil is used for its immune-boosting and stress-reducing properties, and it is often used to treat a variety of conditions, including digestive disorders, respiratory infections, and stress-related disorders. The leaves and stems can be made into a tea, tincture, or oil, and they are often used in combination with other herbs for maximum effectiveness.

While holy basil is generally considered to be safe, it is important to note that it can interact with some prescription medications, including blood-sugar lowering medications, blood thinners, and immunosuppressants.

MEADOWSWEET

Meadowsweet (Filipendula ulmaria) is a perennial herb that is native to Europe and Asia, and it is known for its fragrant and medicinal properties. This herb is a popular addition to a medicinal herb garden, and it is prized for its ability to soothe digestive complaints, reduce inflammation, and provide pain relief.

To grow meadowsweet, you will need to choose a location in your garden that provides full sun to partial shade, and it prefers well-drained soils that are rich in organic matter. Meadowsweet can be propagated from seed or cuttings, and it is best planted in the spring or fall.

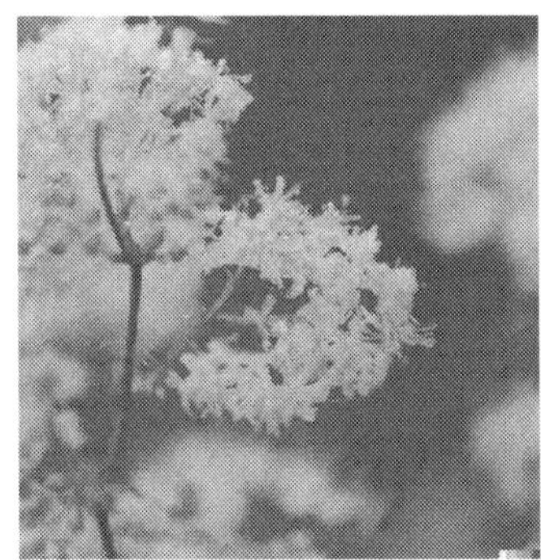

Meadowsweet is used for its anti-inflammatory and pain-relieving properties, and it is often used to treat a variety of conditions, including digestive complaints, headaches, and joint pain. The flowers and leaves can be used fresh or dried to make teas, tinctures, and salves, and they are often used in combination with other herbs for maximum effectiveness.

While meadowsweet is generally considered to be safe, it is important to note that it can interact with some prescription medications, including blood-thinning medications and nonsteroidal anti-inflammatory drugs (NSAIDs).

JIAOGULAN

Jiaogulan (Gynostemma pentaphyllum) is an herb native to China and is known for its adaptogenic properties, which means it can help the body adapt to stress. It is a fast-growing vine that can reach up to 20 feet in length, making it a great option for covering a trellis or pergola.

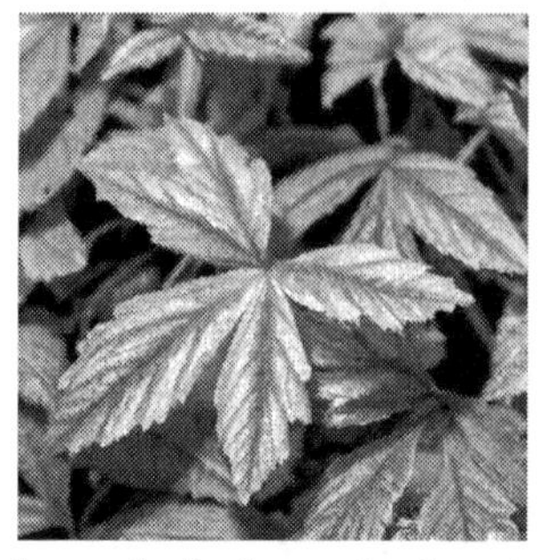

To grow jiaogulan in your medicinal herb garden, it is best to start with cuttings or seeds, as the root system of jiaogulan can be difficult to transplant. Plant the cuttings or seeds in well-draining soil in a sunny location, and keep the soil consistently moist but not waterlogged. Jiaogulan is hardy in zones 7-10, but can also be grown in a pot and brought indoors during the winter in cooler climates.

Jiaogulan has been used for centuries in traditional Chinese medicine to help support the immune system, lower cholesterol and blood pressure, and improve energy and stamina. It can be consumed as a tea, tincture, or capsule, but it is important to speak with a healthcare provider before starting any new supplement or herb, especially if you are taking medications or have a medical condition.

While jiaogulan is generally considered safe, there have been some reports of gastrointestinal upset, headaches, and allergic reactions in some people.

STINGING NETTLES

Stinging Nettles, also known as Urtica dioica, is a common perennial herb that can be found growing wild in many parts of the world. It is a nutritious and medicinal plant that has been used for centuries to treat a variety of health conditions. Growing stinging nettles in a medicinal herb garden is a great way to have a readily available source of this versatile plant.

To grow stinging nettles, start by finding a sunny or partially shaded location in your garden with well-draining soil. Sow the seeds in the spring or fall, covering them with a light layer of soil. Water regularly, especially during dry periods, and keep the area weed-free. Stinging nettles are hardy plants that can withstand cold temperatures and grow well in most climates.

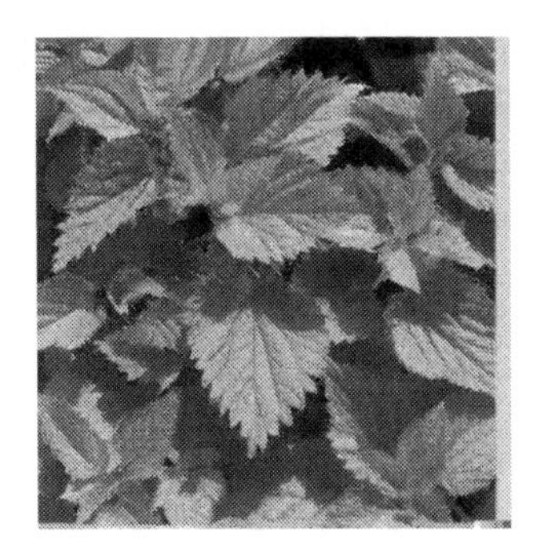

Stinging nettles are commonly used for their anti-inflammatory and pain-relieving properties. They are often made into a tea or tincture to help alleviate symptoms of arthritis, gout, and other inflammatory conditions. Nettles are also rich in vitamins and minerals, including iron, calcium, and vitamins A and C, making them a great addition to the diet for those who are nutritionally deficient.

It's important to note that handling and ingesting raw stinging nettles can cause skin irritation and a stinging sensation due to the tiny hairs on the plant's leaves. Wearing gloves when harvesting the plant or cooking the leaves before consumption can help avoid this. Additionally, people with allergies or autoimmune disorders should exercise caution when using stinging nettles as they may cause an adverse reaction.

SPILANTHES

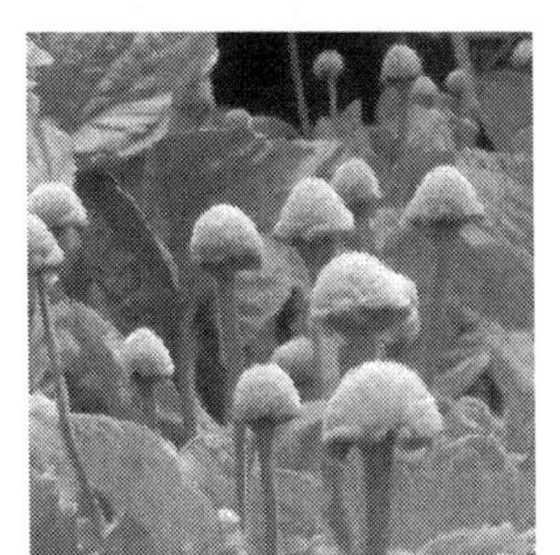

Spilanthes, also known as the "toothache plant," is a medicinal herb that has been used for centuries to treat a variety of ailments. It is a hardy plant that grows well in warm, moist climates, making it an ideal choice for those looking to cultivate their own medicinal herb garden.

To grow Spilanthes, start by selecting a location that has well-drained soil and is exposed to full sun. Once the soil is prepared, plant Spilanthes seeds directly into the ground and keep the soil consistently moist until the seeds have germinated and established a strong root system. It is important to note that Spilanthes does not tolerate frost, so it may be necessary to bring the plants indoors during the winter months in colder climates.

Spilanthes has a long history of use as a natural remedy for toothache and other oral health problems, as well as for digestive and immune system issues. When applied directly to the affected area, the plant's unique compounds help to numb the pain and reduce inflammation. It can also be taken internally as a tea or tincture to promote overall health and wellness.

Despite its many benefits, it is important to be aware of the potential side effects of using Spilanthes. Some people may experience skin irritation or an allergic reaction when applied directly to the skin.

WILD BERGAMOT

Wild Bergamot, also known as Monarda fistulosa, is a hardy and versatile plant that can be easily grown in a medicinal herb garden. This plant is native to North America and is commonly found in meadows, prairies and along the edges of woods.

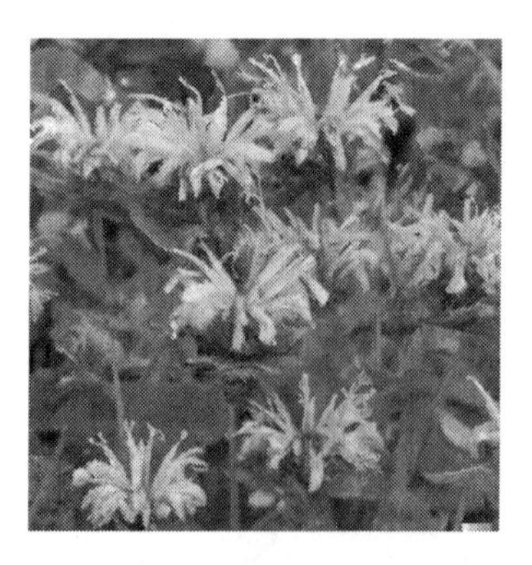

Growing Wild Bergamot is relatively easy, as it is a hardy plant that can adapt to a variety of growing conditions. It prefers full sun and well-draining soil, but can also tolerate partial shade and moist soils. The plant should be spaced about 18-24 inches apart and can be grown from seed or cuttings.

Wild Bergamot is commonly used for its medicinal properties and has been traditionally used for centuries by Native American tribes for various ailments. The plant is rich in essential oils and is used for its antibacterial, antifungal, and anti-inflammatory properties.

Wild Bergamot can be used to treat colds, flu, indigestion, and headaches. It is also commonly used to promote healthy skin, reduce stress and anxiety, and to boost the immune system.

While Wild Bergamot is generally considered safe when used in appropriate doses, it is important to exercise caution when using this plant. The plant contains menthol and other essential oils that can cause skin irritation or allergic reactions in some individuals.

LAVENDER

Lavender is a popular herb that has been used for its medicinal properties for centuries. It is known for its fragrant aroma and is often used in aromatherapy for its relaxing properties. Growing Lavender in a medicinal herb garden is not only easy, but it also offers numerous benefits.

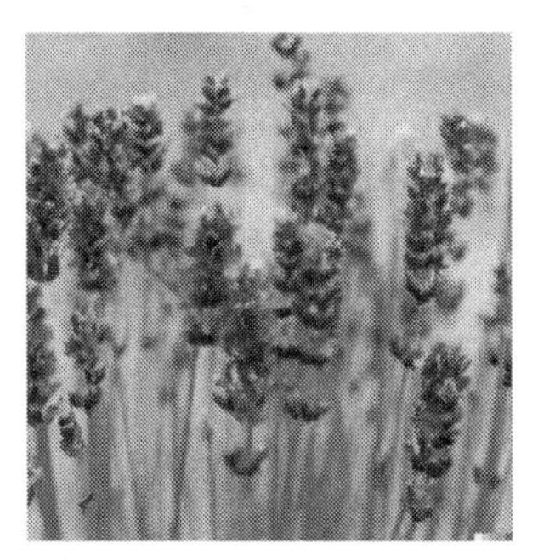

To grow Lavender, select an area with well-drained soil and full sun exposure. Lavender is a hardy herb that is drought-tolerant, so it does not require frequent watering. When planting Lavender, it is important to space the plants out enough to allow for adequate air circulation. This will help prevent disease and improve the overall health of the plant.

Lavender has many medicinal properties that make it a useful herb to have in your medicinal herb garden. It is commonly used as a natural remedy for stress, anxiety, and insomnia. Lavender essential oil can be applied topically or inhaled to help soothe and calm the mind and body. Additionally, it has antiseptic and anti-inflammatory properties and has been used to treat skin conditions such as eczema, psoriasis, and acne.

When using Lavender as a medicinal herb, it is important to keep in mind that it may interact with certain medications, such as sedatives and antidepressants.

CHAMOMILE

Chamomile is a delicate, yet hardy herb that is a must-have in any medicinal herb garden. Chamomile is native to Europe and Asia, but it can be grown in many regions of the world. It prefers full sun to partial shade and well-drained soil. This herb is easy to grow from seed or from divisions of an established plant.

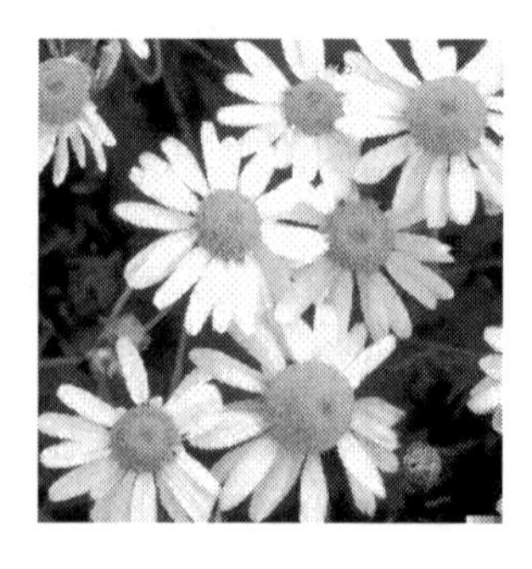

Chamomile is a well-known remedy for its calming and soothing properties, making it an excellent choice for helping with stress, anxiety, and insomnia. The flowers of the plant can be dried and used to make tea, or used as an essential oil in aromatherapy. The tea is especially helpful for aiding in sleep, promoting relaxation, and reducing digestive problems.

In addition to its calming properties, chamomile has anti-inflammatory and antibacterial properties, making it useful for treating skin conditions like eczema, and reducing the symptoms of conditions like colds and flu. It is also believed to have pain-relieving properties and can be applied topically to treat muscle pain and arthritis.

When using chamomile for medicinal purposes, it is important to be aware of any potential side effects. The herb is generally considered safe for most people, but some people may be allergic to it, and it can cause skin irritation when applied topically.

SAGE

Sage is a commonly grown herb in a medicinal garden, known for its strong, pungent aroma and numerous health benefits. It is a hardy perennial that can grow up to two feet tall and prefers full sun to partial shade, well-drained soil, and moderate watering.

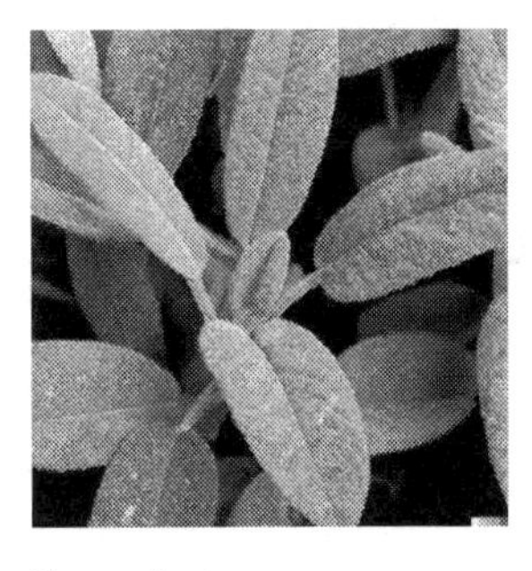

Sage has a long history of use in traditional medicine for its antimicrobial and anti-inflammatory properties, making it a popular natural remedy for a range of health issues including digestive problems, respiratory infections, skin irritations, and mental fatigue. It can be used in a variety of forms, including dried leaves for tea, essential oil, or as an infusion in oil or vinegar.

For pain relief and to reduce inflammation, sage can be applied topically in a salve or used in a hot compress. It can also be used as a mouthwash to soothe sore gums and mouth ulcers. Inhaling sage essential oil is said to help improve cognitive function and alleviate stress and anxiety.

While sage is generally considered safe when used as directed, excessive use can cause irritation to the mouth and throat, as well as nausea and dizziness.=

ST. JOHN'S WORT

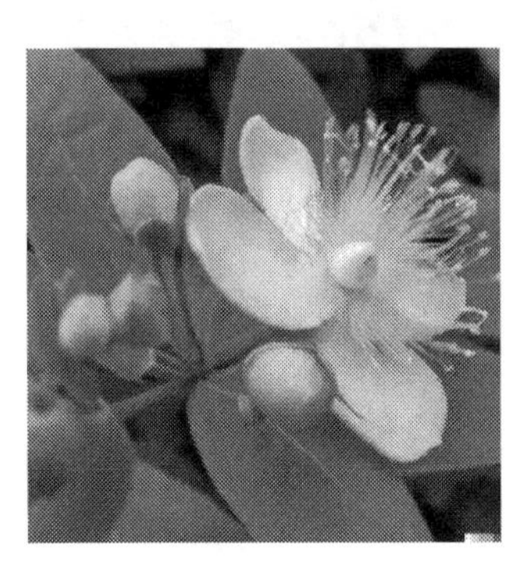

St. John's Wort, sometimes referred to as "nature's Prozac", is a popular herb that is often used for its potential mood-lifting and anti-anxiety effects. Growing St. John's Wort in a medicinal herb garden is easy, as the plant prefers well-drained soil and full sun to partial shade.

To grow St. John's Wort, start by purchasing seeds or young plants from a reputable supplier. The seeds can be sown directly in the ground or in containers. Once established, the plant will grow to be about 2-3 feet tall, with yellow, star-shaped flowers that bloom in the summer.

St. John's Wort is commonly used for mild to moderate depression, anxiety, and insomnia. It is also sometimes used for nerve pain, attention deficit hyperactivity disorder (ADHD), and other conditions, but more research is needed to confirm its efficacy for these uses.

It is important to note that St. John's Wort can interact with certain prescription medications, such as antidepressants, birth control pills, and others.

VALERIAN

Valerian is a perennial flowering herb that is native to Europe and Asia, and has been widely cultivated in many parts of the world. With its long history of use as a medicinal herb, Valerian is a great addition to any medicinal herb garden. To grow Valerian, plant the seeds in well-drained soil in a sunny or partially shaded location. The plant prefers moist soil and does best in a slightly acidic soil. It is a hardy plant that requires minimal care once established, making it a great option for those who are new to growing medicinal herbs.

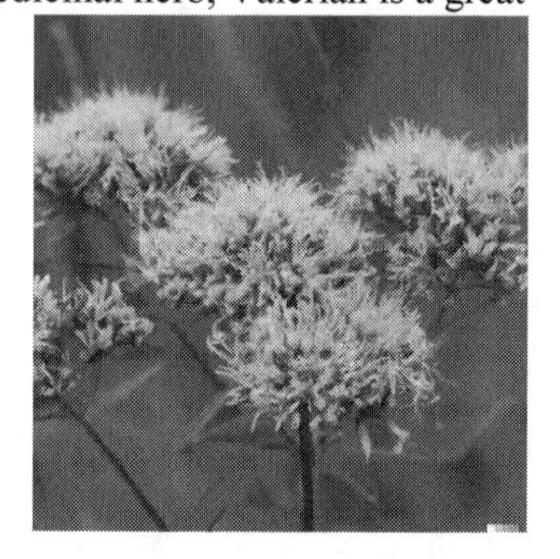

Valerian is commonly used as a natural remedy for sleep disorders, anxiety, and stress. It has a calming effect on the body and mind, which makes it a popular choice for those who are looking for a natural way to relieve anxiety and improve sleep quality. Valerian can be taken as a supplement in the form of capsules, tablets, tinctures, or teas. The root of the plant is the most commonly used part and is considered to be the most potent part of the plant in terms of medicinal properties.

While Valerian is generally considered safe, it can cause some side effects in some individuals. Some people may experience gastrointestinal side effects, such as bloating, gas, or diarrhea, when taking Valerian.

CATNIP

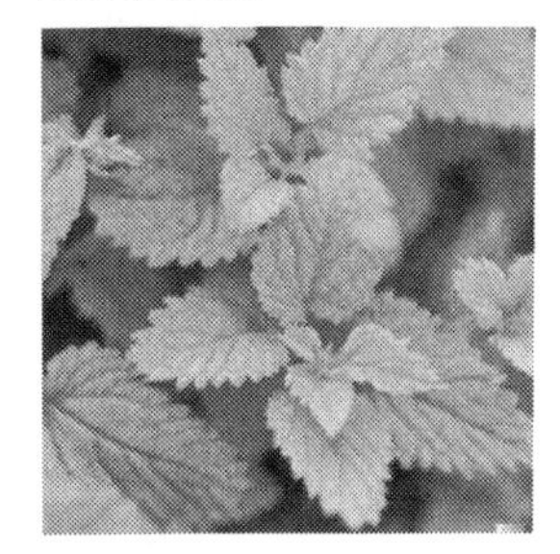

Catnip (Nepeta cataria) is an easy-to-grow perennial herb that can be found in many herb gardens. It is best grown in well-draining soil in a sunny location and can reach up to three feet in height. The plant is known for its fragrant, lemon-scented leaves and tiny white or pale pink flowers that bloom in the summer.

Catnip is often used for its calming and relaxing effects on cats, but it also has medicinal properties for humans. It has been used as a natural remedy for digestive issues, headaches, and insomnia. The leaves and stems of the plant contain compounds that act as mild sedatives, making it useful for relieving anxiety, stress, and promoting sleep.

To make a tea, simply steep a handful of fresh or dried catnip leaves in boiling water for 10-15 minutes, then strain and enjoy. It can also be taken in supplement form, such as capsules or tinctures, but it's important to follow the recommended dose to avoid any potential side effects.

However, it's important to note that not everyone may be able to use catnip for medicinal purposes. Pregnant or breastfeeding women should avoid catnip as its effects on these populations are not well known.